Restorative Flow Yoga

Giving something back to the body that works so hard for you.

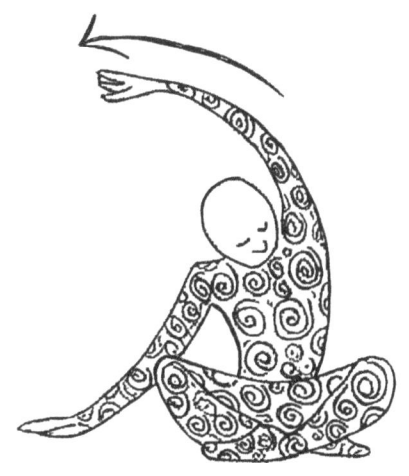

By Donna Belk

Cover and book design by Donna Belk.
Printed in the United States of America.

ISBN-13: 978-1512117851
ISBN-10: 1512117854

8.5" x 11" (21.59 x 27.94 cm)
Black & White on White paper
148 pages
BISAC: Health & Fitness / Yoga

Contents

View short video clips of the poses being demonstrated online at
www.donnabelk.com/restorativeflow

Introduction

Restorative Flow Yoga is a luxurious practice that encourages students to slow down and notice the subtle changes that occur within. Restorative Flow Yoga classes offer a deep nourishing experience which activates the body's natural healing abilities.

A Restorative Flow Yoga practice differs from restorative poses in that restorative poses take quite a bit of time to set up and use a lot of props. Of course, they are worth the effort! The restorative poses are also held for extended times, sometimes as long as 10-15 minutes. Many yoga teachers have said that they would like to offer restorative yoga, but don't want to haul all the props around with them.

In Restorative Flow Yoga, the postures are done one after the other in gentle flowing movements. A sticky mat and a blanket are the only props a student needs. This makes it easy for yoga teachers who go from one site to the next to teach their classes to offer this style without having to tote lots of blankets, blocks, etc.

This training will be useful to you as a yoga teacher because it will add to your repertoire of yoga methods. And the Restorative Flow Yoga poses can be used in your regular hatha yoga classes to warm up, to create a more gentle class, or to cool down before savasana. Going into savasana from these Restorative Flow Yoga sequences really deepens the savasana experience for students.

Who are the students for this style of yoga?
* those who want to deeply relax
* elders, seniors
* those with illnesses such as fibromyalgia, chronic fatigue syndrome, arthritis
* those dealing with the effects of stress
* those with limited range of motion
* those wanting a contemplative practice
* yoga teachers who want to add a specialty to their yoga class offerings
* yoga teachers wanting to incorporate Restorative Flow Yoga into their regular hatha yoga classes

How this style differs

* No corrections—you can't do it wrong in Restorative Flow Yoga. There is no right way to do a pose, only the way that feels pleasurable.
* Keep people in feeling state, not mental thinking processes: few instructions, quiet times with no talking
* Restorative Flow Yoga is pleasurable. Pleasure catalyzes the relaxation response, promoting parasympathetic dominance, and full digestive force, full healing (repair) of body.
* The poses are presented in an a la carte fashion. Do a whole class with the poses, intersperse a few into your regular classes, use them as warm ups or cool downs.
* Although they look peaceful, restorative poses can be challenging to the mind.

Advantages of Restorative Flow Yoga

Restorative Flow Yoga poses help relieve the effects of chronic stress in several ways (this happens naturally)
- Breath is slowed down
- Paying attention to the internal body
- Body is doing relaxed, rocking motions
  - Studies have shown that rocking alleviates many stress-related conditions (high blood pressure, anxiety, disorientation, tension, depression) and reduces pain. Ex: Nursing home residents who rocked were both happier, and healthier, and requested less pain medication
  - It has been very well documented that a gentle repetitive motion has a soothing and calming effects (think babies, and Russian treatment of out-of-control people—they used to teach this in American nursing but don't so much anymore). This affords rapid relief of stress and tension.
  - Rocking facilitates gentle, rhythmic contraction and relaxation of back muscles which results in a stronger and more limber spine and joints
  - Stimulates blood flow and this helps improve circulation and cell oxygenation (stimulates the autonomic nervous system to open the bronchioles). With this movement of blood comes enhanced exchange of oxygen and waste products so toxins are released from the body.
  - Gently manipulates the internal organs
  - Improved lymphatic drainage
  - It improves the sense of balance by stimulating the body's ability to maintain balance
  - Relieves lower back pain (JFK had rocker in the Oval Office)
  - Polarity therapy has rocking around the joints, Trager massage, Thai massage
  - Working with the "ether" element in the body
  - Sensory integration
  - Subtle energy
  This movement is found as Kundalini flows up the spine, and is present in Quakerism, Shakerism, Judaic davening (torso-rocking prayer), whirling dervish of Islam, Goddess-worshipping circle dance, flowing movements of tai chi, estatic shamanic dance, middle eastern belly dance, and bioenergetics
    - Mimics the natural rhythms of the body – heart squeezes and releases, digestion occurs by this tightening and release motion,
    - Doing pose in motion is easier for some people

Relaxation Scripts

Following are two relaxation scripts you may use in your class. They can be used at the start, or at the end of your class.

Green Mist Relaxation

And breathe in, and breathe out, and begin to relax. If your hands are crossed, uncross them. If you have your body constricted so that circulation is cut off, notice this. Allow your body to say to you what it needs in order to be comfortable in this time and space. Even if it seems like an odd thing that the body is asking of you, try it. And then later if that need changes, change again. It is fine. The body is the holder of the now. It is a very, very important part of your experience of this thing you call life. Cherish it and recognize its sacred needs. And if your eyes have not lowered, lower or close them gently. And breathe.

Now imagine that in the center of this space, begin to sense a tiny, tiny dot of Green Mist. And at first it is a tiny dot you can tell that as it begins to spin, as it begins to spin, it is like a beautiful ball growing and it's filled with Green Mist. And as the Green Mist expands and grows, you can see it begin to fill this space. Soon you can feel it at the bottoms of your feet. You can tell that it is ready to come inside.

As it touches your feet and finds the magical portal, it begins to enter through the bottoms of your feet. And as it enters you can feel it surrounding the outside, and swirling inside, and your feet are relaxed. And as the mist continues to swirl and move and expand and grow, it moves up, up into your ankles, into your shins. And you can feel it on the outside of your legs and on the inside of your legs, and they relax. And as the Green Mist continues to grow and expand, it reaches your knees. And you can feel it on the outside, and you can feel it on the inside. And as the Green Mist continues to expand, and as the Green Mist continues to grow, you can feel it on the inside of your upper legs, you can feel it on the outside. And your legs, your whole entire legs relax. And as your Green Mist continues to expand and grow, it moves into your hips. Your hips relax. All tension is gone. And the Green Mist continues slowly to move up your torso, both inside and outside, and you can feel each vertebra in your back relax – like someone beautifully playing a musical instrument and as each note is touched the back relaxes.

And the Green Mist continues to expand and grow and it swirls inside and outside the torso, it reaches the shoulders. And the shoulders relax. And the Green Mist goes down the upper arm, into the elbows, the forearms, inside and outside the Green Mist travels, into the hand, and each finger and the hands, and the arms relax. All tension is gone. And as the Green Mist continues to expand and grow it moves into the neck, and the neck relaxes. So long it's had to work holding up the head, and now it can relax.

And the Green Mist continues to grow and expand and the jaw relaxes. The area around the mouth relaxes. The eyes relax. The nose relaxes. The face, the head, the ears, all relax. All tension is gone. And as the Green Mist continues to swirl and grow, the entire form is relaxed, and this entire space is filled with relaxation.

—long pause—

And returning to this place of the Green Mist. And noticing that the Green Mist also has movement about it, a joyfulness as it begins to contract. You can feel it going over the outside of your face, and inside your face. You can feel its magnificence as it leaves you with tickles of joy. And it moves down through the neck area, comes up from your fingers and hands and arms, through your shoulders. And down your torso the Green Mist travels leaving behind wonderful feelings of peace and joy. Into the hips, relaxing the hips, upper legs, into the knees. Down the legs the Green Mist travels leaving relaxation behind. Into the ankles, into the feet. The soles of feet feel wonderfully relaxed, and exiting through the magical portal at the bottoms of your feet.

—long-pause—

And gathering itself up into a tinier and tinier ball in the center of the space. And know that the Green Mist is always there for you. You have but to think the phrase "Green Mist" and you can recall it to yourself, and instantly you'll remember the wonderful feelings as they soothe all your energy lines, as they soothe your form.

—pause—

And returning fully to this space and this time knowing that you are relaxed. You are ready for whatever is ahead of you. In this moment you have found the resources that you have always wanted to be all that you are. And wiggling your fingers and wiggling your toes, gently begin to allow yourself to return to this time and space. And be very gentle and slow with yourself. Coming back.

Progressive Relaxation Inquiry
[Read slowly, add pauses in as you read]

Allow yourself to rest comfortable and breathe normally. There is no need to hurry or to do things the "right" way. Simply relax back, and breathe comfortably at your own pace and rhythm. There is no hurry, nothing to do except be in the moment right here, right now. If your thoughts wander, that is fine, as much as possible simply bring your noticing back to the rhythm of your breath.

Can you notice the air as it brushes against your nostrils as you inhale? And, can you feel the warmth of the air against the back of your throat as you exhale? Simply notice.

Is there any tightness or clenching in the jaw? If yes, gently, gently, let it go. Just as much as is possible in this moment. And even noticing the tongue, is it pressed against the roof of your mouth? Or is it resting comfortably on the floor of your mouth?

Does your chin feel like it is jutting up towards the ceiling, or can you elongate the back of your neck and head for a more comfortable positioning? It's ok to move, you don't have to hold perfectly still. Wiggle, make micro adjustments as needed so you're comfortable. And only you know what comfortable feels like.

What about your forehead? Does it feel smooth or are you furrowing your brow?

Even your ears … can you relax even your ears back and down?

And your shoulders, do they feel like they are raised or hiked up towards your ears? Or can you relax them down and back?

Gently, gently, let everything go as much as is possible. The breath is long and slow, deep and smooth, soft and easy.

Are your arms comfortable, or can they be adjusted so they can relax even more? Does it feel better if your palms are up facing the ceiling, or turned down? Or even resting on your belly? What is most comfortable for you here in this moment, just for now?

No right or wrong answers, simply what is most comfortable for you here and now.

Bring your attention to the right hand, the wrist, the back or top part of your hand, the tip of your thumb, index finger, middle finger, ring finger, pinky finger, the palm of your hand, and back to your wrist.

And your left hand, the wrist, the back or top part of your hand, the tip of your thumb, index finger, middle finger, ring finger, pinky finger, the palm of your hand, and back to your wrist.

Relaxing, and letting go.

Noticing the heart area of the chest. Can you soften around the heart? And think of the heart relaxing back and down. Inhale and softly exhale "Ahhhhhh" to your heart.

The belly soft and full. Noticing the rise and fall of the belly as you inhale and exhale. Allow your attention to ride on top of the belly for a breath or two as the belly rises up and softly descends with each inhale and exhale.

Ahhhhhhhh, gently, gently, letting go. Softening the belly.

Noticing the lower back. Is it comfortable? Do you need to bend your knees to be even more comfortable? It's ok to wiggle and readjust. Whatever it takes to enhance your comfort is fine. You can't do it wrong.

If your legs are straight, then letting them rest heavy against the floor . There's no holding or supporting you need to do right now.

And bring your attention to the feet, and softening even the feet. And notice the ankle of the right foot, the top of the right foot, the tip of the big toe, second toe, .third or middle toe, fourth toe, pinky toe, the bottom or sole of the right foot., the heel, and back to the ankle.

And the left foot, the ankle of the left foot, the top of the left foot, the tip of the big toe, second toe, .third or middle toe, fourth toe, pinky toe, the bottom or sole of the left foot., the heel, and back to the ankle.

If you want to, just for the fun of it, pretend that you are breathing in and out through your whole body, from the top of your head to the bottoms of your feet. Inhaling from your feet, clear up to the top of your head and back down again.

Gently resting, softly breathing, letting go. And here, pausing in silence for a moment.

[Silence for 2 minutes]

Slowly, slowly, coming back. Noticing the body and sending your appreciation to the body for the movement and mobility it gives you. Slowly, gently beginning to move fingers and toes, and wiggling in any direction the body wants. There's no hurry.

And when you're ready, ever so slowly, making your way up to a comfortable seated position.

Breathing Practices

Corpse pose
- Observe the rise and fall of the abdomen at the navel center.
- Observe and eliminate jerkiness.
- Be aware of, and eliminate pauses.
- Gently allow the breath to slow down naturally.
- Allow breath to be so smooth that it is quiet.
- Imagine energy of breath is flowing up and down the spine.

Qualities of breath
Look for these qualities in your breath Say one quality on the inhale, the next on the exhale, etc.

"We want the breath to be long, and slow. Deep and smooth. Soft and easy. Quiet, and even."

Alternate Nostril breathing
Exhale and inhale from one nostril five times. Then, do five times with the other nostril. That is called a "round." Doing three rounds is a complete practice.

Gradually, begin to do this with attention, not the fingers, allowing attention to move from one to the other nostril. One sits quietly, with eyes closed, and simply places attention on the nostril.

Ujjai breathing
In Ujjai breathing, the throat is partially closed and it sounds like you're whispering with your mouth closed. You can also feel a flow of air on the palate. A slightly different sound is heard on inhalation and exhalation. During inhalation, one tightens the abdominal muscles very slightly, and during exhalation the abdominal muscles are used to exhale completely. One feels the air and listens to the sound during the practice.

Spinal breathing
There are a variety of practices with awareness moving up and down the spine with the breath. One may do this practice between particular energy centers (chakras) or form different shapes of the visualized flow, including elliptical or a figure-eight.

The most straight forward method is to
- Imagine the breath flowing from the top of the head, down to the base of the spine on exhalation, and to
- Imagine the flow coming from the base of the spine to the top of the head on inhalation.

- This may be done lying down, or in a seated meditation posture.

One may simply experience the breath, or may be aware of a thin, milky white stream flowing in a straight line, up and down. This practice is very subtle when experienced at its depth, and can turn into a profoundly deep part of meditation practice.

Teaching Techniques

The following teaching techniques are used to make the Restorative Flow Yoga class relaxing for the students. These techniques support the participant's ability to relax, and the poses themselves take that relaxation even further. If you are not teaching Restorative Flow Yoga simply use these techniques to further your own ability to relax within the poses.

Intention

Intend that the class be slow and gentle

As a teacher you set the pace and tone of the class. If you're calm, peaceful and relaxed that will be communicated to your students just by your presence, without you having to say or do anything. Use this to your advantage! Begin class in an unhurried, gentle way. Take a moment to breathe before you begin and be clear about your deepest intent in teaching the class. Ask yourself, "Who am I as a yoga teacher," and, "What do I want to convey?"

Restorative yoga is not yoga therapy

A restorative class is for relaxing, reducing stress, and allowing the body's own natural healing capabilities to engage. Restorative yoga, is <u>not</u> therapy. It is important that your students don't think you are going to prescribe or diagnose or treat their ailments. Rather than offering solutions when students tell their yoga teachers about their ailments, it is more empowering for the student if the yoga teacher encourages them to investigate their own solutions. Certainly yoga teachers can suggest different postures, or variations but ultimately it is up to the student to listen to their own body wisdom.

Voice characteristics

How a teacher uses her voice in class can have a profound impact on students. Our voices communicate just through their pitch, tone and timber. A lower-pitched voice is more relaxing to students. A slow-paced voice communicates calmness. We can impact the students in our class just by the *sound* of our voice!

Voice low and relaxed

Keep your voice low and relaxed during class and practice this when you're alone so it becomes comfortable to you. It's proven that the lower your voice pitch, the more authoritative you sound. A lower voice is also more psychologically pleasing to people.

Speak slowly

If your mind is thinking very quickly, "What posture are we going to do next? What are other details I need to tell students?" then you might unconsciously speak quickly. The pace of your voice reflects the state of your mind. In a restorative class there is lots of permission to add in the suggestion to breathe. If you find your thoughts running away with you, tell students to breathe while you think ahead a posture or two. Then when you're ready to resume teaching you can relax knowing that you're prepared to teach the next several postures.

Soothing, rocking tone of voice
What do we mean by a rocking tone of voice? Try this experiment: say the words "up and down" in a sing-song voice. You probably lifted the tone of your voice on the word "up" and lowered your tone on the word "down." This rocking or up-and-down tone is soothing to students and reinforces the rocking and circular motions of Restorative Flow Yoga. It can even create memories to people of a time when they were children and adults spoke to them in a sing-song voice.

Sighing helps students relax
Hearing the teacher sigh helps students relax, it is like a yawn that is contagious. The "ahhhhh" sound creates a strong physical reaction in people. You can usually see students visually relax if, as the teacher, you take a breath yourself and exhale it with an "ahhhh." If you feel awkward about this ask someone to do this for you so you can see the impact it has on you physically. If you feel positively about it, then please give that gift to your own students.

Atmosphere

Maintain a quiet atmosphere
Maintaining a quiet atmosphere helps enhance the nurturing, relaxing and soothing qualities of the class. It is also easier for students to turn their attention inward if they are not distracted by loud sounds.

Dealing with noises in class
If you know there will be noises (people coming in late, fitness equipment clanging in the next room, another class letting out before yours, etc.) give the instruction for students to allow any sound to pass through them as if they were transparent. Also tell students, "Any sounds you hear only help to relax you more deeply." Or, "Welcome all sounds into your experience."

Allow quiet times in class with no instruction
Stop talking for periods of time throughout the class. A pause of two or three minutes is fine. Many instructors have so much to say about the poses that class time is filled with talking. Having quiet pauses helps the students notice the sensations of their body more deeply. After you ask a question, such as, "Can you feel the sensation along the side of your neck?" be especially careful to allow 10 seconds or so of quiet so the student can reflect on the answer.

Eliminate filler words such as "uh, er, ah." Eliminate advanced filler words such as "really, just, so." Eliminate filler phrases such as "You're gonna," and "I want you to."

Verbal cues

Ask students to notice internal sensations
When an instructor asks the students to notice sensation in their body it helps keep their focus on their internal feelings vs. the mechanics of the posture. An example of an inward-asking statement is, "Follow your breath as it makes its way down into your lungs."

Encouraging students with verbal cues
In many yoga classes so much emphasis is put on the precision of the posture that students are anxious about whether they're doing the posture right. It helps students relax if the teacher assures them that they are not doing anything wrong.

Here are some suggested phrases for teachers to say to convey that to students:
> "slow and easy – there's no hurry"
> "you're doing good"
> "excellent"
> "you can't do it wrong "
> "nice job"
> "that was great"
> "good, good, good"
> "go at your own pace"

Help students relax with verbal cues
Verbally encouraging students to relax gives them permission to go more deeply into the pose. However, if you tell someone to relax they sometimes don't know how, or where to begin. Following are some phrases to use rather than just saying "relax."
- o "everything is loose and easy"
- o "loosen the jaw, drop the shoulders"
- o "sink downward"
- o "gently, gently let go"
- o "release downward"
- o "let gravity do your work for you"
- o "let your scalp drop back"
- o "melt into the mat"
- o "relax open"
- o "ride the wave of your movements"

Cue in advance
Most students like to know what they are going to be doing next or how long they are going to be holding a posture. Try to give students a few seconds notice before changing from one pose to the next. This creates safety so students can relax even more, and neurologically it prepares mind and body for what you're going to do next.
- o "one or two more times, and then pausing"
- o "continue the pose in motion to the rhythm of your own breath"
- o "… and when you're ready, coming back to center for another breath or two"
- o "allow yourself about 10 more seconds"
- o "two or three more breaths and in your own timing coming back to sitting"

Postures

Use postures that can be done on the floor, limit number of standing postures
It is more relaxing if students stay in a seated, prone or supine position on their mats rather than coming up to standing and back down to seated. Many people are rest-deprived and not having to get up and down is a welcome relief.

Use postures which circle the joints, or rock the body
Postures which circle the joints or rock the body are instinctively soothing to the body. A person naturally rocks an infant or child as a way to comfort them. Rocking chairs have been around for centuries, and people who are traumatized naturally rock in an effort to find solace.

Rocking is calming to the entire body and is especially beneficial to the lymphatic system since muscular movement is what helps move lymph throughout the body. Forward-bending is also calming to the nervous system and promotes inner reflection.

Breath

Begin the class with a breath awareness meditation or noticing of the breath
Beginning the class with breath awareness helps students relax immediately. Breathing practice will also take their attention inward. Breath is a theme that weaves through all restorative yoga classes. It's one of the most potent tools we have as yoga teachers.

Integrate the breath with all postures
It helps students relax more if the breath is integrated into the smooth flow of class. Give breath instruction for every pose, especially those postures that are done in motion. Also, give permission for students to breathe at their own pace rather than trying to do it "right." Their natural breath should always be honored over a particular breathing pattern. If a student's natural breath flows and works with specific breathing patterns that is great! If it does not, it is more comfortable for the student to breathe at their own pace.

Sustained poses

Hold postures 2-10 minutes, or translate that into breaths such as, "Hold for 10 deep breaths."
By holding or sustaining poses, it allows the student to relax more deeply into the pose and also physically allows the muscles to release open *if* the student is comfortable. Usually the mind wanders after a few seconds when postures are held, so in sustained postures cue students occasionally to bring their attention back to the sensation of the stretch or to their breath.

Cue students how long you're going to hold pose so they feel safe and know how to pace themselves
If students know they have two or three minutes to maintain a pose they can pace themselves as they move through the pose. It is also relaxing to the student to know what to expect next as it diminishes their anxiety about being prepared for the next move. Reassure students by saying, "I'll measure the time for us."

Supported poses

Use of props
Standard props for a yoga class include blankets, blocks, chairs, straps, sandbags, etc. A yoga rule of thumb seems to be the more props the better. However, teachers that teach in many locations do not have the ability to travel with a lot of props. Be creative in using the props that may be on hand in the locations where you teach. For example, if you are teaching in a corporation's conference room, use available chairs. If you are teaching in a gym, use 1 or 2 pound weights as sand bags. Know that whenever you use props it disrupts the smooth flow of a class because you have to get the prop and either demonstrate or give instructions on how to use it. Also, the goal of a restorative class is not necessarily to go more deeply into a pose but to relax into openness. If you feel that the student can be encouraged by the use of a prop, then by all means, use one.

Also consider these props
- eye pillows
- music is soft and gentle
- philosophical readings (religious readings can make some students feel uncomfortable)

Passive poses
Encourage students to release all muscular tension so the pose is completely passive. Most yoga teachers can observe where students carry tension in their bodies and make suggestions to them individually or as a group about what areas to relax more deeply. Even if students *think* they are releasing muscular tension, a teacher's observations can be beneficial to them. Please make suggestions to individual students quietly so they don't feel pointed out or embarrassed.

Stress and Tension

Signs of tension
Following are common areas where students hold tension in their bodies:
- holding the breath
- furrowing of the brow or forehead
- shoulders that seem lifted up
- clenched jaw or pursed lips
- clenched hands
- relaxed hand with one or two fingers lifted
- hand or foot tapping

Rushing through the movements
Students may have a tendency to rush through the movements because they are simple poses and appear easy to do. The speed at which people move is very telling about the state of their mind, which is one of the reasons why students are encouraged to move slowly in Restorative Flow Yoga. When students are asked to notice the sensations of their bodies it slows things down for them because they turn inward with their thoughts. You can draw your students' attention inward by asking questions, or by cueing them. An example for cueing torso circles is: "Let one complete inhalation and exhalation equal one complete circle of the torso. Inhaling as you circle back, and exhaling as you circle forward." An example of a question is, "Where does the sensation occur in your hips?"

Create a nurturing environment

Here are some ideas for creating a nurturing and safe environment:
- welcome students warmly when they come in
- begin and/or end class with singing bowls, bells, gongs
- cold stone to place on forehead
- essential oils, a drop placed on forehead or under nose to those not sensitive to scents (dilute oil so it doesn't burn the skin)
- flowers
- warm room
- low light
- incense and candles (be aware, some people are sensitive to fragrances and would not find them relaxing)
- careful touch such as Reiki or Healing Touch
- offer to put blankets over students if they are cold at the end of class
- assure students you'll be watching over them during savasana so they can let go completely
- tell students that you'll be around for a few minutes after class if they want to talk

Healing

Yoga has very powerful healing properties. I believe that most yoga teachers become teachers because they want to offer the healing aspect of yoga to other people. Following are some important points to remember as a yoga teacher.

- Healing does not necessarily mean that someone is going to get better. Illness can have many gifts to it and can be a great teacher.
- You do not want to interfere with anyone's life path, or anyone's course of learning, or anyone's way.
- In creating a safe, restful environment you allow students to open their hearts and experience the divine love which is by nature who they are. This is tremendously healing and impactful.
- Our body naturally moves toward health and healing. The "medicine" is within us.

Benefits of the poses

One of the techniques for creating a deeply relaxing class is to keep the focus of students on the sensations of their body. If the teacher is giving detailed instructions on how to do the poses or citing the purposes of the poses, this can keep the students in their thinking mind rather than on the sensations of the body.

Following are general health benefits of the poses in this workbook.

Circular motion poses
- o the gentle activity of the body's muscles accelerates the blood's circulation of oxygen and nutrients
- o blood pressure is lowered by the slow relaxed pace
- o brain wave frequency decreases which is associated with many self-healing responses
- o deep breathing supports relaxation
- o deep breathing causes the diaphragm to descend and compress the lymph-rich tissues of the organs and glands. This propulsion of lymph carries toxins out of the body as well as carrying the immune cells throughout the system.

Twisting and bending poses
- o exercises the muscles along the spine which in turn stimulate the nerve reflexes along the spine that activate the organs and the connective tissue that holds the spine together
- o movement massages the contents of the intervertebral disks toward the center of the disk itself, which helps to sustain the bulk of the disk in spite of gravity's downward pull. This also helps maintain a healthy distance between the vertebrae, which allows enough room for the exit of nerves from the spine
- o expands and compresses the sides of the rib cage, helping to increase or maintain the flexibility of the ribs and the capacity to expand the rib cage in breathing
- o organs are compressed then released causing the propulsion of lymph within them which helps to eliminate waste products, cleanses the tissues, and enhances the function of the organs

Relaxation benefits
- o reduces pressure within the circulatory system by expanding the size of the capillaries which helps to prevent strokes, and reduce the risk of circulatory problems
- o increased size of blood vessels allows for most effective delivery of blood rich in oxygen and nutrition into the tissues, organs and glands
- o all diseases – cancer, heart disease, metabolic disease, anxiety, depression – are improved with relaxation practice
- o the beauty of these simple movements is that they allow the mind to have a focus and this helps keep the mind free from worries and complexities
- o deep relaxation is not far from meditation and prayer. Quite a bit of research has demonstrated that relaxed, focused intention that we call meditation or prayer has significant effect.

RESTORATIVE FLOW YOGA POSES

Standing Poses

View short video clips of the poses being demonstrated online at
www.donnabelk.com/restorativeflow

Circle all the Joints

Moving into the pose
- from a standing position go through the body circling all the joints 5-10 times in one direction and then the other direction
- circle the ankles one foot at a time
- squeeze the toes together and separate the toes as far as you are able
- circle the knees (feet hip-width apart, or feet together)
- circle the hips
- circle the shoulders
- circle the elbows
- circle the wrists
- squeeze the hands into fists and then separate the fingers as far as you are able
- circle the neck or roll head from side to side
- circle the eyes
- circle the tongue in the mouth, gathering saliva and then swallowing it

Breath
- breath is easy and natural

Fine points
- pace is slow and easy
- eyes are closed or resting downward

Inquiry
- "As you circle the joints, are there areas where you have no sensation? Or where you can't feel the movement?"

Subtle energy (think about, pretend, imagine)
- create space in all the joints, encircling them with softness and warmth

Effect
- calming

Benefits
- cues nervous system and mind to be present

Teacup Hands

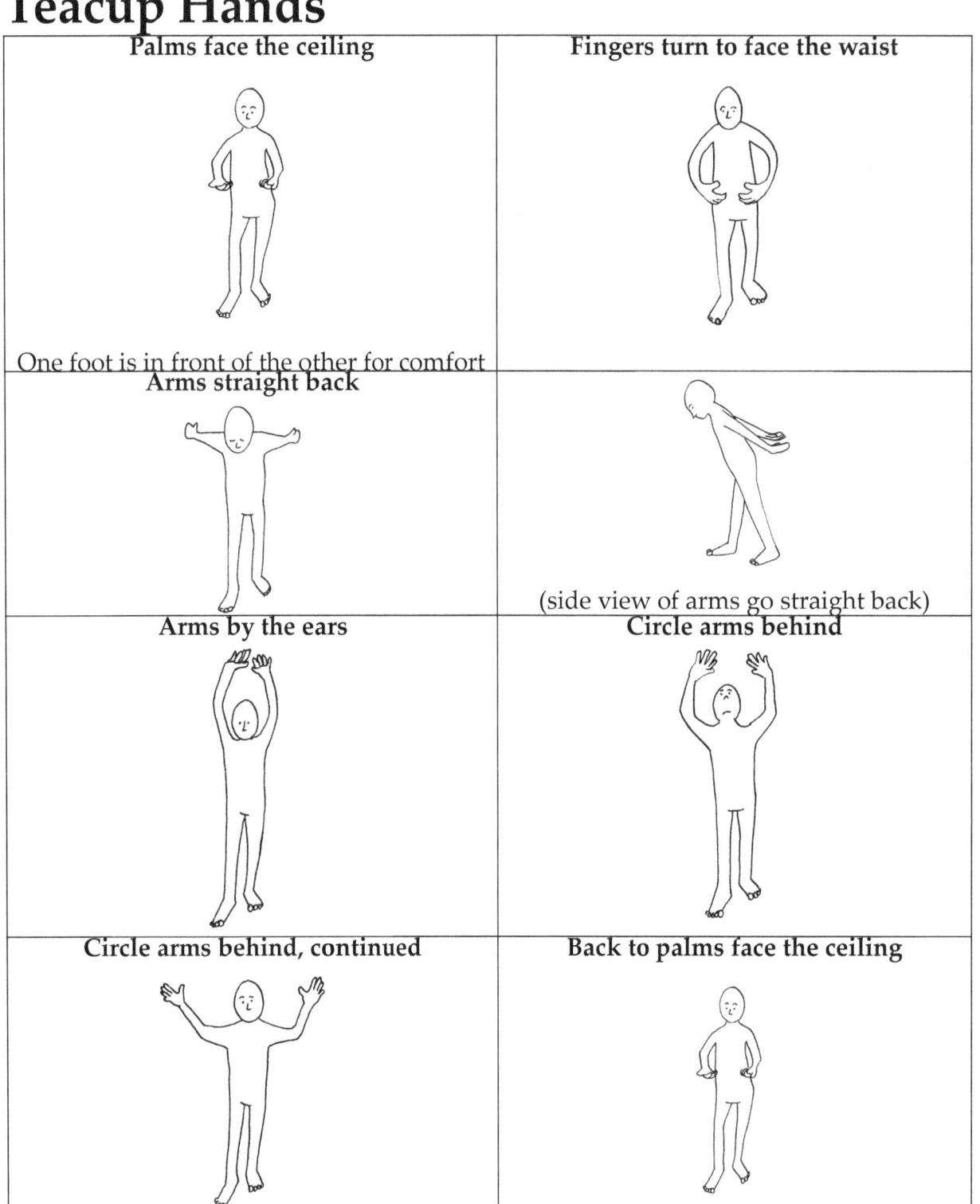

Palms face the ceiling

Fingers turn to face the waist

One foot is in front of the other for comfort

Arms straight back

(side view of arms go straight back)

Arms by the ears

Circle arms behind

Circle arms behind, continued

Back to palms face the ceiling

Forward and Backbending of the Spine

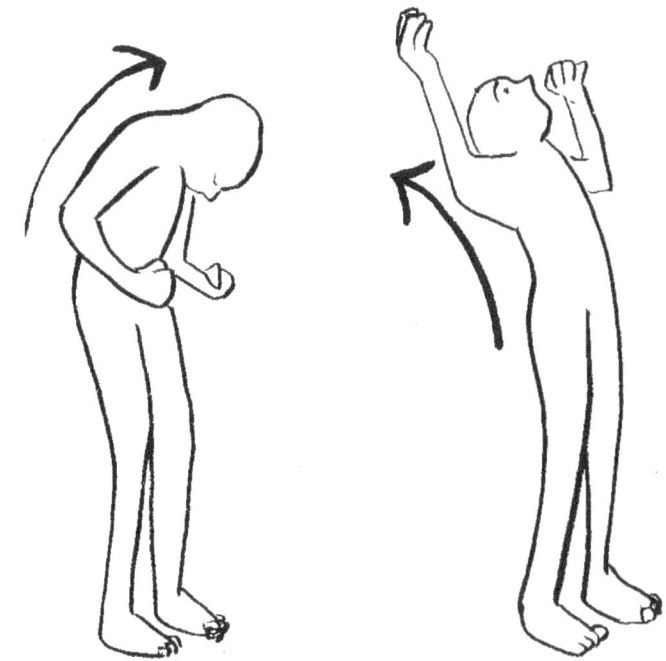

Moving into the pose
- standing with the feet about hip-width apart
- make fists with your hands and curl forward, chin touching the chest, drawing the belly button toward the spine, furrow the brow and tighten the jaw
- relax the fists, face and belly and arch back slightly lifting the arms to fully open the chest
- continue the movement curling forward and arching back

Breath
- breath is easy and natural
- to apply the breath to the movement inhale as you arch back and exhale as you curl forward

Fine points
- knees are slightly bent
- tense the body as you curl forward, relax the body as you open back
- pace is slow and easy
- eyes closed or resting downward

Variations
- this can be done in a chair

Inquiry
- "Are there areas that seem difficult to relax?"
- "Is it easier for you to tense muscles, or relax them?"

Subtle energy visualization
- the chest opens and closes like a flower
- send energy out through hands, pull it toward you on contraction
- contract into pearl or dot of light behind the navel

Effect
- expansive and contractive

Benefits
- limbers the spine
- massages the axillary area where lymph nodes are located helping them distribute lymph throughout the body
- strengthens ability to balance
- strengthens arches, calves, quadriceps
- contraction provides lots of sensation so it is good pose for people who want to gain more body awareness
- develops concentration and focus
- massages the internal organs

Flying Tadasana

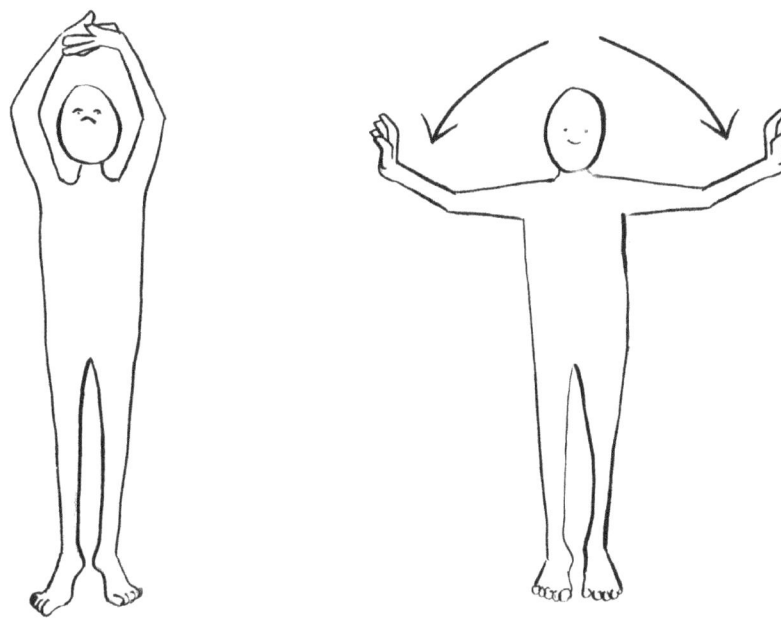

Moving into the pose
- begin with the feet separated about hip width apart
- lift the arms overhead and at the same time come up so you're standing on the toes
- return the arms to the starting position and the feet to the floor at the same time

Breath
- breath is easy and natural
- inhale as the arms lift and you come up on your toes, exhale as the feet return flat to the floor and the arms come down

Fine points
- stretch is gentle and easy
- try to coordinate the movement so that you're feet return to the floor at the same time the hands return to the sides of your body
- keep the knees slightly bent for better balance rather than stiffening the legs when you're on your toes

Variations
- bring the arms up like a bird lifting for flight, bring hands in prayer position overhead and as you come down bring the hands straight down the center of the body
- while standing on the toes, lift one foot from the floor
- with the arms overhead and the feet flat on the floor stretch one side of the body and then the other by reaching with the arms

Inquiry
- "As you lift your arms during the inhale, can you feel your chest expand and your breath deepen?"

Subtle Energy
- drawing up earth energy, when hands meet at top drawing down heavenly energy; as hands float down, rainbow colors extend from the fingertips

Effect
- expansive

Benefits
- lifting of the arms assists in breathing into the deepest areas of the lungs
- strengthens ability to balance, combining grace and balance at the same time
- strengthens the arches, ankles, and legs
- develops concentration and focus

Lift the Arms and Lift the Toes

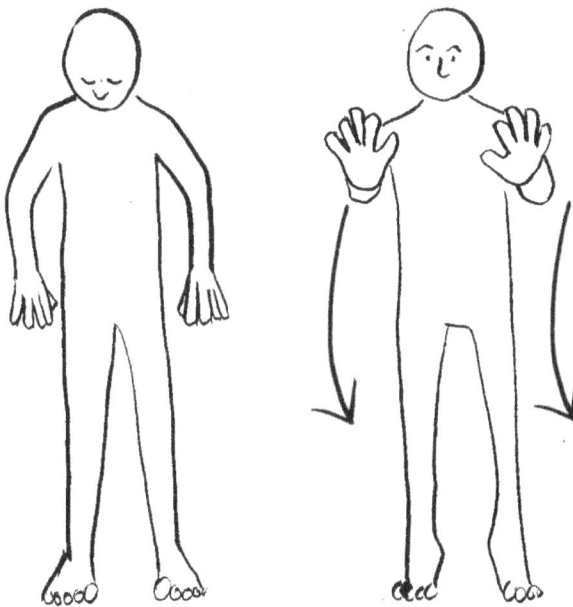

Moving into the pose
- standing with the feet separated about hip-width apart
- slowly come up onto the toes and at the same time lift the arms to about shoulder-height, then return so the feet are flat on the floor, arms are alongside the body, then lift the toes

Breath
- breath is easy and natural
- inhale as you lift to your toes and the arms come up to shoulder-height, exhale as the feet return flat to the floor and the arms come down

Fine points
- pace is slow and easy
- elbows point toward the floor
- knees, wrists and elbows are slightly bent during the entire movement
- eyes are resting downward
- as you lift arms first the wrists rise, then the knuckles and then the fingers

Variations
- when you lift the toes balance on the heels of the feet
- when you come up on the toes, lift one foot so you are balancing on only one leg

Inquiry
- "Are your arms relaxed, or are they stiff?"
- "Are you knees locked, or are they slightly bent?"

Subtle energy visualization (think about, pretend, imagine)
- fingers are long and rake through the earth as they come down

27

Effect
- balancing, harmonizing, soothing, calming, focusing

Benefits
- massages the axillary area where lymph nodes are located helping them distribute lymph throughout the body
- strengthens ability to balance, combining grace and balance at the same time
- strengthens arches, ankles and legs
- develops concentration and focus

Easy Triangle

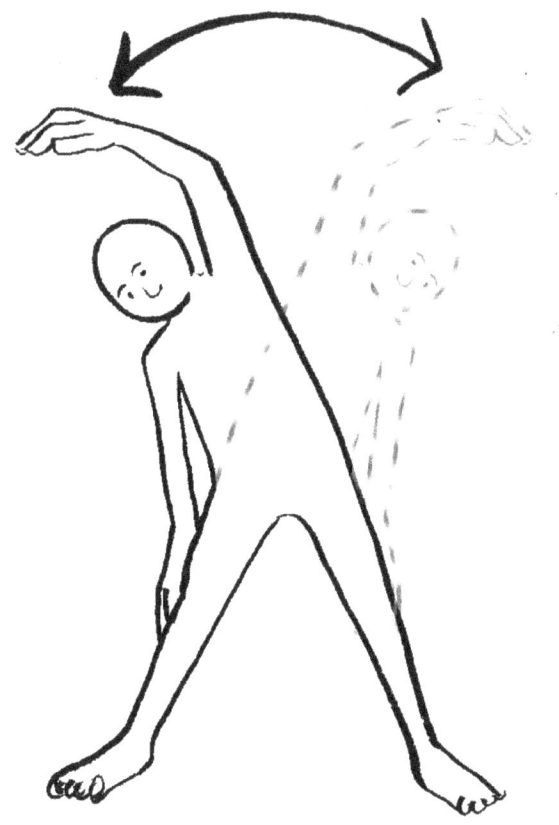

Moving into the pose
- feet are slightly wider than hip-width apart
- bring one arm above the head so the arm is by the ear
- slide the other arm down the side of the leg bending as far to the side as you are able
- come back to center and repeat on other side, and continue flowing from one side to the other

Breath
- easy and natural
- exhale as you bend to the side, inhale as you come back to center

Fine points
- pace is slow and easy
- eyes are looking downward

Variations
- hold the pose on one side rather than doing it in motion
- keep hands over heart as you bend from side to side

Inquiry
- "Can you feel the stretch along the side of the torso?"
- "Can you feel from your hips to the fingertips?"

Subtle energy visualization (think about, pretend, imagine)
- with hands over heart, you are being rocked in the arms of a loved one
- as you rock to one side, the foot sinks into the earth about 4 feet

Effect
- soothing, harmonizing

Benefits
- lateral movement for the spine helps to increase awareness and spaciousness between the ribs
- limbers the spine
- helps maintain flexibility of ribs and capacity to expand the rib cage in breathing

Horse Stance

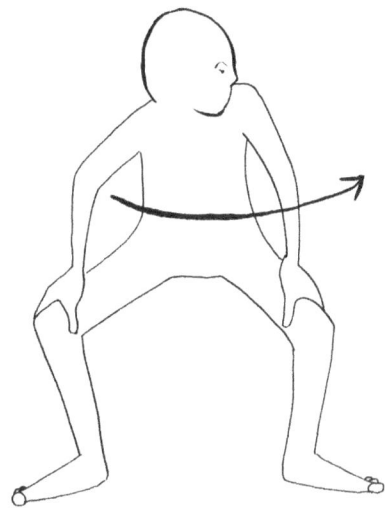

Moving into the pose
- separate the feet about 3' apart
- bend the knees
- hinge at the hips bending forward
- bring both hands to rest above the knees
- bring one shoulder into the center, and turn to look behind the other shoulder
- switch to the other side
- continue the movement flowing from one side to the other

Breath
- breath is easy and natural
- inhale as you come to center, exhale as the you turn to the side to look behind

Fine points
- pace is slow and easy
- bend the knees as deeply as is comfortable
- fingertips can be facing each other, or turned away from each other
- first turn at the base of the spine, then the mid- and upper-back, then the shoulders, and lastly turn the head and eyes

Variations
- hold the pose on one side rather than doing it in motion

Inquiry
- "Where is the most sensation for you in this pose? Neck, shoulder, inner thigh, legs, or back?"
- "As you return to center each time, do you naturally want to inhale or exhale with the breath?"

Subtle energy visualization (think about, pretend, imagine)
- energy spirals up the spine like a barber pole and with each spiral prayers are being sent out like a Buddhist prayer wheel

Effect
- grounding, balancing

Benefits
- opens the hips and shoulders
- limbers the spine
- massages internal organs

Windmill

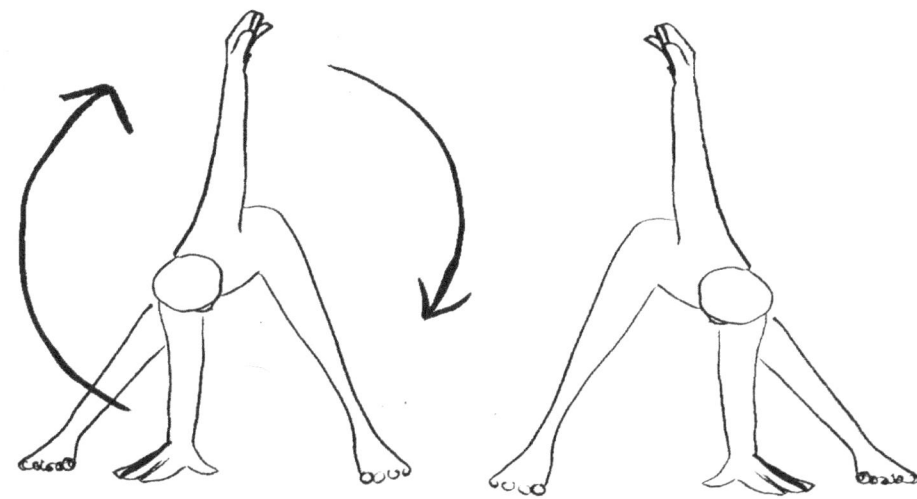

Moving into the pose
- separate the feet about 3' apart
- hinge at the hips bending forward
- bring both hands or fingertips to the floor with the face looking at the hands
- keep one hand on the floor and look at the back of the other hand
- keep your eyes on your hand and lift the hand to point toward the ceiling
- still keeping your eyes on your hand return the hand to the starting position
- switch to the other side
- continue the movement flowing from one side to the other

Breath
- breath is easy and natural
- inhale as the hand reaches toward the ceiling, exhale as the hand returns to the floor

Fine points
- pace is slow and easy
- bend the knees if necessary for comfort
- eyes follow the hands during the entire movement (as long as it feels good)

Variations
- hold the pose on one side rather than doing it in motion
- glide your hand along your belly to show your belly how to rotate rather than rotating from the shoulder

Inquiry
- "Can you notice a twisting motion in your spine?"
- "Does it feel better to your body to exhale as the hand reaches toward the ceiling rather than inhale? Or inhale as the hand returns to the floor?"

Subtle energy visualization (think about, pretend, imagine)
- energy spirals up the spine like a barber pole
- when hand lifts toward the ceiling you are extending your compassion and appreciation to the world

Effect
- grounding, balancing

Benefits
- opens the back of the legs
- limbers the spine
- massages internal organs
- helps neck move through full range of motion

Poses All Fours

View short video clips of the poses being demonstrated online at
www.donnabelk.com/restorativeflow

Cat & Cow *Marjariasana*

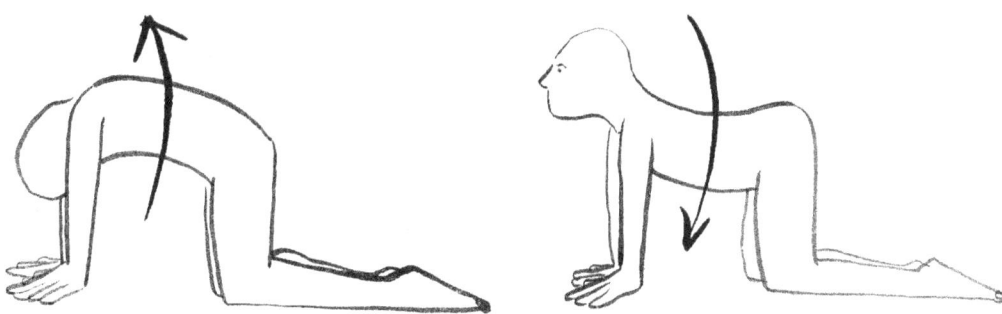

Moving into the pose
- come to an all fours position
- tuck the chin in toward the chest and arch the back as if you were an angry cat
- look towards the ceiling and let the belly be soft as if it were a hammock
- continue the pose in motion at your own pace

Breath
- breath is long and slow
- exhale as you tuck the chin into the chest and inhale as you lift the face to look toward the ceiling

Fine points
- pace is slow and easy
- knees are underneath the hips, wrists are underneath the shoulders
- knees are about hip-width apart, hands are about shoulder-width apart
- toes can be flat or toes can be curled under
- when arching the back like a cat think of drawing the tip of the nose toward the pubic bone
- if there is discomfort in the wrists then make the hands into fists, or put a small towel under the wrists, or come to rest on the elbows

Variations
- extend one arm and the opposite leg parallel to the floor; on an exhale bend the arm and leg as if to touch one another, on the inhale reach out again stretching diagonally
- cow circles
- wag the dog's tail
- your tail bone is a paintbrush and you have four brush sizes; start with the smallest paint brush size and circle the tailbone to the largest brush size

Inquiry
- "Can you feel the sensation from your belly button to your chin as you look toward the ceiling?"
- "Can you feel a stretch along the back of your body as you tuck the chin to the chest?"

Subtle energy visualization (think about, pretend, imagine)
- an energy ball rests on top of the sacrum and as you move the ball rolls up the spine and then back down again
- the sun is shining down on the spine warming it

Effect
- expansive and contracting

Benefits
- limbers the spine
- massages internal organs

Thread the Needle

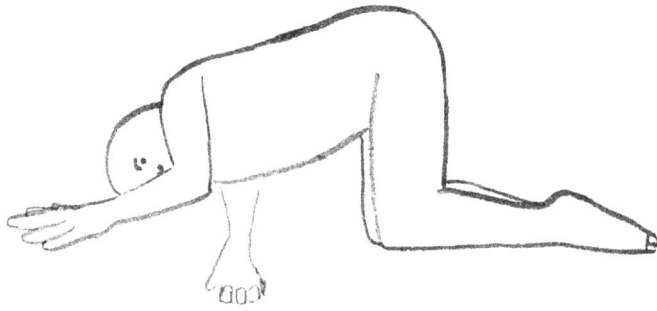

Moving into the pose
- from an all fours position
- take the right hand and slip it underneath the body below the left wrist
- reach as far as you can with the right hand until the shoulder comes down to the floor
- allow the head to also rest on the floor as much as possible
- hold for 1-2 minutes

Breath
- breath is long and slow

Fine points
- stretch is gentle and easy
- head may rest on the floor
- pick the supporting arm up off the floor and let it rest naturally where it wants (flop it!)
- as the hand slides underneath the body to create the stretch there are three hand positions that can be used,
  - hand slides underneath the body by the wrist of the other hand
  - hand slides underneath the body by the knee
  - hand slides underneath the body midway between the hand and the knee

Variations
- for a flowing sequence sink back into child's pose between each variation
- turn the chest toward the ceiling

Inquiry
- "How deeply in your shoulder can you feel?"
- "Can you distinguish any of the tendons or ligaments that are so numerous in the shoulder girdle?"
- "Think of the range of motion you have with the shoulder joint, and what that range of motion allows you to do."

Subtle energy visualization (think about, pretend, imagine)
- follow the line of energy from deep within the shoulder to the center of the palm of your hand, and then back and forth; follow the line of energy from the elbow to the palm of the hand, and then back and forth
- follow energy from sacrum up the spine and send it out through the center of the palm of your hand; also send out energy through each finger as if there were ribbons of energy coming from them

Effect
- calming

Benefits
- opens the shoulder
- limbers the spine

Child's Pose (cradling the face) *Balasana*

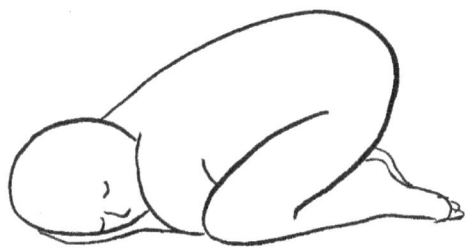

Moving into the pose
- from an all fours position sink the hips back toward the feet into child's pose
- from child's pose tuck the elbows in between the knees
- palms turn to face the ceiling
- lower the head and turn the face to the side so the head rests in the palms of your hands
- think of loving hands, as if you were holding the face of a child you loved
- hold for 1-2 minutes

Breath
- breath is long and deep

Fine points
- stretch is gentle and easy
- the tailbone drops toward the floor
- chin is tucked
- if there is any discomfort in the knees straighten them a bit or come into a prone relaxation pose

Variations
- separate the knees and feet for a marvelous inner thigh stretch

Inquiry
- "Can you feel the ribs move in the back of your body as you inhale and exhale?"
- "Which direction does your tailbone move as you exhale? Which direction does your tailbone move as you inhale?

Subtle energy visualization (think about, pretend, imagine)
- the energy is spiraling inward as if you were in a cave filled with sparkles and twinkling lights
- massage the internal organs with warmth, light or sound

Effect
- comforting, soothing, calming

Benefits
- allows the spine to relax completely
- calms the nervous system
- allows the internal organs to relax fully

Moving Child's Pose

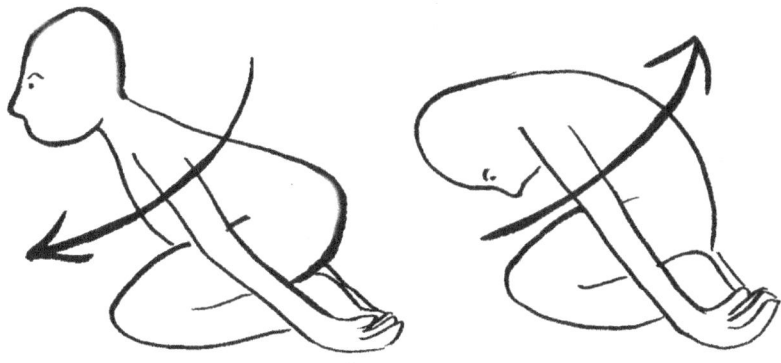

Moving into the pose
- from an all fours position sit back on your feet so you torso is upright
- draw the shoulder blades together and lift the chest to the ceiling as you arch back
- allowing the arms to be very relaxed
- slowly hinge forward from the hips folding as far forward as you are able
- when you have reached your maximum fold, round the back and slowly curl up to an upright position again
- continue the pose in motion at your own pace

Breath
- breath is long and deep
- (variation 1) exhale as you hinge forward and inhale as you return to center
- (variation 2) inhale as you swan dive forward, and exhale as you roll up to center

Fine points
- pace is slow and easy
- arms are hanging at the sides, they are not engaged in any movement

Variations
- place tops of feet flat on the floor or curl toes under
- if there is any discomfort in the knees then do not bend them as much or come into a comfortable seated position

Inquiry
- "Can you allow your arms to completely relax, or do they engage as you go through this movement?"

Subtle energy visualization (think about, pretend, imagine)
- the chest opens and closes like a flower
- contract into pearl or dot of light behind the navel as you come up

Effect
- expansive and contractive

Benefits
- limbers the spine
- massages internal organs

Seated Poses

View short video clips of the poses being demonstrated online at
www.donnabelk.com/restorativeflow

Circle the Joints

Moving into the pose
- from seated position systematically go through the body to circle the joints
head (stimulates the thyroid)
shoulders
elbows
wrists
fingers
squeeze the hands into fists and then separate the fingers as far as you can
circle the eyes
circle the tongue in the mouth, gathering saliva and then swallowing it
- 3 to 5 times in one direction, pause, then reverse directions

Breath
- breath is easy and natural
- to apply breath to the movement, exhale as you circle forward, and inhale as you circle back

Fine points
- pace is slow and easy
- when circling the head be cautious not to let the neck just hang back; instead keeps the neck elongated by lifting the chin to the ceiling as the head circles back
- eyes can be closed or resting

Variations
- for the hands, make the hands into fists squeezing them tight, then open the hands as wide as the fingers can stretch
- for the hands, press the thumb and index finger together and squeeze as tight as you can; next place the middle thumb and middle finger together, and continue through all the fingers
- for the wrists, make figure eight movements with the hands
- a flowing pattern is to circle the shoulders-elbows-arms, and repeat this pattern several times

Inquiry
- "How deeply can you feel into the joint?"
- "Can you notice the ligaments and tendons of the joint?"

Subtle energy (think about, pretend, imagine)
- encircling the joints with warmness, like honey
- sparkles of light or colors swirling in the joints

Effect
- calming

Benefits
- cues nervous system and mind to be present
- moves all joints through their full range of motion
- excellent method for increasing subtle body awareness

Torso Circles

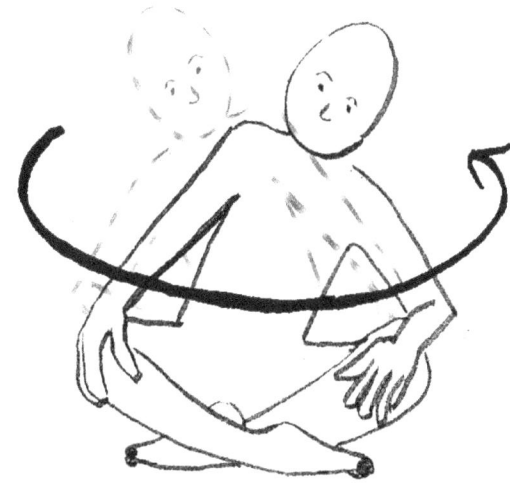

Moving into the pose
- from a comfortable seated position rest the hands on the knees
- hinge forward from the hips and begin to circle the torso
- 5-7 times in one direction, pause, then reverse directions

Breath
- breath is easy and natural
- exhale as you circle forward, and inhale as you circle back

Fine points
- back is elongated
- chin is slightly tucked
- eyes closed or resting

Variations
- if sitting with the legs crossed is uncomfortable, then students may sit with one or both legs straight
- add head/neck circles as you rotate the torso

Inquiry
- "As you circle around 360 degrees, are there areas where you have no sensation?"

Subtle energy visualization (think about, pretend, imagine)
- swirl the energy within the body like when you swirl a mug and the contents swirl on their own accord after you stop swirling the mug

Effect
- harmonizing, calming

Benefits
- limbers the hips and spine
- moves the hips through their full range of motion

Seated Triangle

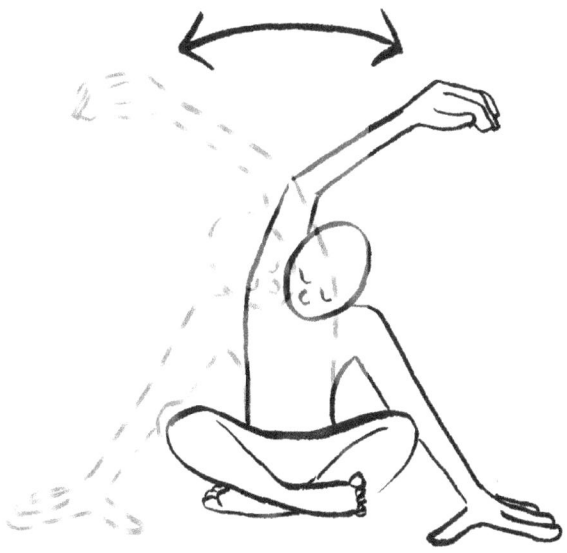

Moving into the pose
- from a comfortable seated position, place one hand on the floor a foot or so away from the hip, and the other arm by the ear
- bend the arm on the floor and hinge to the side as far as you can go; come back to center, switch arm positions and repeat on the other side
- continue the pose in motion, going from side to side

Breath
- breath is easy and natural
- exhale as you bend to the side, and inhale as you come back to center

Fine points
- the arm on the floor can be straight, with the elbow gently bent, or it can be bent with the forearm resting on the floor
- the arm by the ear can be straight, with the elbow gently bent
- both sit bones remain on the floor
- chin can be tucked, or tucked then turned toward the ceiling

Variations
- hold on each side for 3 to 5 breaths rather than doing the pose in motion
- place hands over the heart as you move side to side

Inquiry
- "Can you feel the stretch from the hip all the way up the arm to the little finger?"

Subtle energy visualization (think about, pretend, imagine)
- light comes from the fingers creating a cocoon of light or energy around you
- if you are holding hands over the heart, imagine you are being rocked in a cocoon of love

Effect
- soothing, harmonizing

Benefits
- lateral movement for the spine helps to increase awareness and spaciousness between the ribs
- limbers the spine

Seated Cobra / Seated Cat Cow

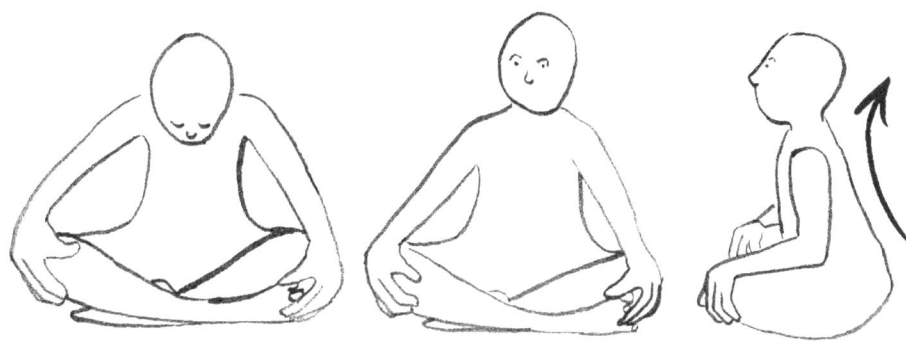

Moving into the pose
- from a comfortable seated position, place the hands on the knees
- on the inhale, extend through the spine and gently arch back lifting the chest to the ceiling and thinking of pulling up out of the hips, and squeezing the shoulder blades together
- on the exhale, draw the chin to the chest, round the back forward, and tuck the tailbone
- continue the pose in motion at your own pace

Breath
- breath is long and deep
- exhale as you curl inward and inhale as you arch back

Fine points
- pace is slow and easy

Variations
- hold the arched back pose a few breaths by resting the hands on the floor by the hips or slightly behind the hips
- inhale spread the arms and exhale hug yourself
- hands on feet and trace circles around body with fingertips
- same arm motion as Forward and Backbending of the spine

Inquiry
- "Can you feel the belly button draw toward the spine as you exhale and tuck the tailbone?"
- "Can you notice the ribs the back of your body as tuck inward?"
- "Can you notice how the sternum lifts toward the heavens as you arch back?"

Subtle energy visualization (think about, pretend, imagine)
- the heart opens and closes as you move back and forth

Effect
- expansive and contracting

Benefits
- limbers the spine
- massages internal organs

Easy Seated Forward Bend

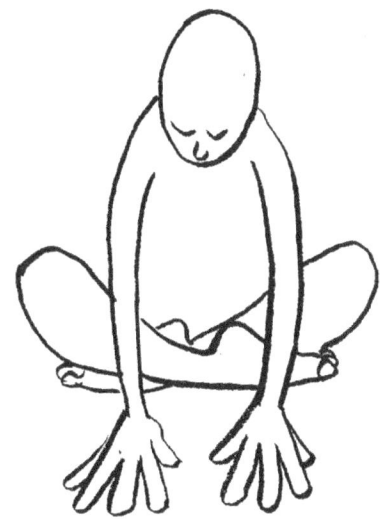

Moving into the pose
- from a comfortable seated position, lengthen through the spine
- hinge forward with the hands or fingertips on the floor in front of the body, reaching as far forward as is comfortable
- hold for 2-5 minutes
- come back to center, reverse the position of the legs and repeat on other side

Breath
- breath is easy and natural
- exhale as you hinge forward and inhale as you come back to center

Fine points
- stretch is gentle and easy
- back is elongated
- chin is slightly tucked
- allow the head to hang forward

Variations
- hold hands in prayer position with elbows resting on knees
- arms can be bent with the head hanging forward, or the forehead can rest on the hands depending on the level of flexibility

Inquiry
- "Can you feel the stretch in your back as you hinge forward?"
- "How far down your back can you feel the sensation?"

Subtle energy visualization (think about, pretend, imagine)
- circle a ball of light, energy or sound in the belly behind the navel
- begin at the sacrum and draw a pinpoint of light, or an image of a pearl, up to the top of the head and back down again; repeat up and down the spine

Effect
- reflective, going inward
- soothing and calming (IF the pose is comfortable for the student to hold)

Benefits
- opens the hips
- calms the nervous system

Easy Seated Twist

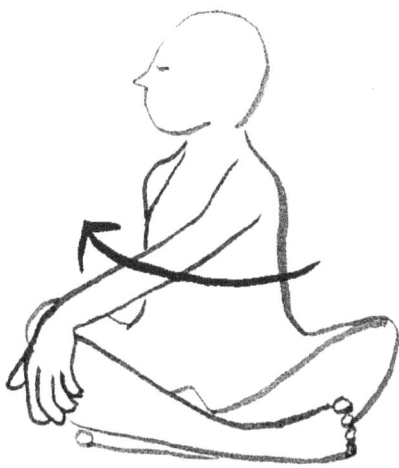

Moving into the pose
- from a comfortable seated position, elongate through the spine and turn to the right placing the left hand on the right knee or thigh, the right hand rests comfortable on the floor beside or behind you
- lengthen through the spine again and exert slight pressure on the left hand as you turn to look behind you even further
- come back to center and repeat on other side
- continue the pose from side to side at your own pace

Breath
- breath is easy and natural
- exhale as you turn to look behind, and inhale as you come back to center
- think of lengthening the spine on the inhale, and twisting a little bit further on the exhale

Fine points
- stretch is gentle and easy
- spine is elongated
- chin is tucked
- shoulders are dropped away from the ears

Variations
- pose can be done with the legs tucked to the same side rather than sitting in a cross-legged position
- float arms up about shoulder-height and then down to touch the earth as if you're coming in for a landing
- windmill arms

Inquiry
- "Can you feel the stretch from the small of your back into the base of your spine?"
- "As you twist from one side and then the other, can you find your center?"

Subtle energy visualization (think about, pretend, imagine)
- spirals of energy start in the spine and rise toward the top of the head and then beyond
- as the hands circle around the fingers graze the edge of a healing pool of water
- draw a circle of light to surround you as the hands circle around

Effect
- harmonizing, calming

Benefits
- limbers the spine
- massages internal organs to help release stored toxins
- helps to release tightness in the lower back

Stir the Pot

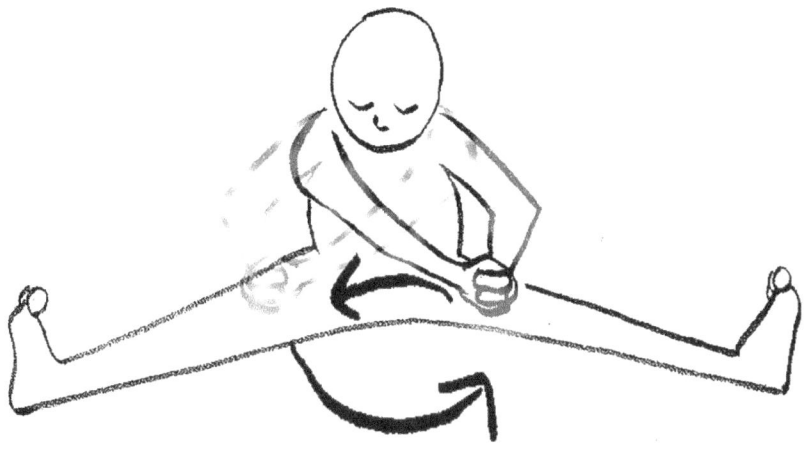

Moving into the pose
- from a comfortable seated position separate the legs into a "v" position
- lengthen through the spine
- clasp the hands and begin to rotate the hands as if you are stirring the outside edges of a big pot of soup
- 3 to 5 times in one direction, pause, then reverse directions

Breath
- breath is easy and natural
- exhale as you circle forward and inhale as you circle back

Fine points
- stretch is gentle and easy
- chin is tucked
- pace is slow and easy

Variations
- extend through the heels for more stretch through the legs
- windmill the arms by touch the toe with the opposite hand
- when hinging forward as far as you can reach, release the hands to the floor and hold for several breaths

Inquiry
- "Can you feel the stretch in your legs as you hinge forward?"
- "As you circle the body 360 degrees, is there any area where the sensation seems to disappear?"
- "Are there areas where you feel intense sensation?"

Subtle energy visualization (think about, pretend, imagine)
- in front of you rest the different components of your life; mix them together so they are smooth and harmonious
- a spoon or stirrer enters through the top of your head and stirs the entire contents of your body

Effect
- soothing

Benefits
- limbers the hips
- gentle stretch for the inner thighs
- strengthens core muscles

Moving Seated Forward Bend

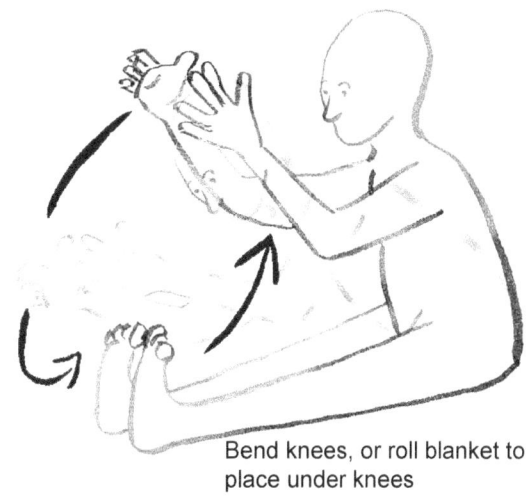

Bend knees, or roll blanket to
place under knees

Moving into the pose
- from a comfortable seated position, bring the legs together stretched out in front of the torso, knees slightly bent
- on an inhale, lift both arms up reaching toward the ceiling
- on an exhale, hinge at the hips and reach both arms toward the feet
- continue the pose in motion at your own pace

Breath
- breath is easy and natural
- exhale as you hinge forward and inhale as you come back to center

Fine points
- pace is slow and easy
- eyes are closed or resting downward

Variations
- straighten the legs if you want more stretch along the back of the legs
- for the knees to be more comfortable, bend them, widen the legs or place a blanket under the knees

Inquiry
- "Do any emotions come up for you as you hinge forward?"

Subtle energy visualization (think about, pretend, imagine)
- you are holding an energy ball between your hands; it enters through the top of your head and you guide it all the way down your body and out the feet; as it leaves your body anything that is out of harmony, or no longer serves you easily flows away. Reverse directions of the energy ball bringing the things into your body that you want and will serve and enhance your life
- as arms reach up gather heavenly energy which is shimmery, and light; as the arms come down the body guide the heavenly energy through your body

Effect
- expansive, calming

Benefits
- stretches the back of the body

Animal Stretch

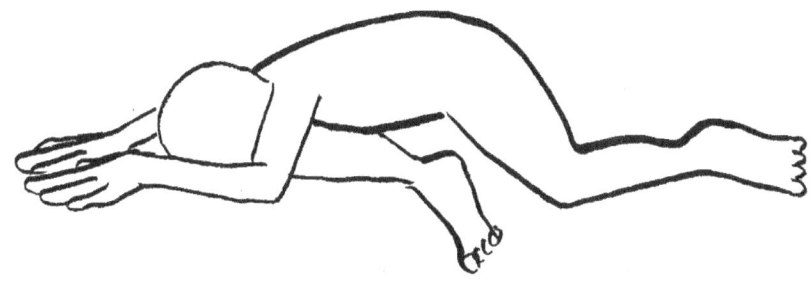

Moving into the pose
- from a cross-legged seated position, keep one foot in front of you, and bring the other leg and foot behind you
- turn so you face the knee of the bent leg that is in front of you
- hinge forward placing your hands on either side of the knee in front of you and resting your torso as much as possible on the thigh so that the bent knee is in the center of the chest by the heart
- the hands can rest beside the bent front knee, or the forearms can rest on the floor
- hold for 2-5 minutes
- come back to center, reverse the position of the legs and repeat on other side

Breath
- breath is easy and natural

Fine points
- stretch is gentle and easy
- chin is tucked
- head is relaxed forward and down resting on the floor or on the hands (make fists with the hands to support the head)

Variations
- turn the belly button towards the floor; place the forehead on the floor with the arms outstretched
- move extra belly flesh to one side out of the way so you can bend forward with more ease
- remain partially upright resting on the forearms
- for more stretch bring the front foot away from the body
- straighten the leg behind for more intensity

Inquiry
- "Can you feel sensation in your hip?"
- "Can you notice how the breath moves the back of your body as you inhale and exhale?"

Subtle energy visualization (think about, pretend, imagine)
- a soothing hand rests on your head or back
- your back is being massaged by hundreds of tiny fingers that know just the right areas to touch

Effect
- calming, soothing, nourishing, focusing

Benefits
- allows the spine to relax completely
- soothes the nervous system
- massages the ascending and descending colon which aids digestion

Gathering Breath

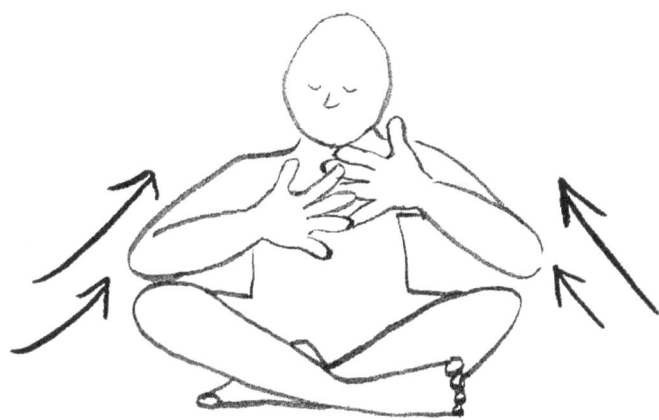

Moving into the pose
- from a comfortable seated position, gently reach your arms forward as if you are gathering or scooping a bouquet of flowers bringing them toward your face as if to inhale their fragrance
- continue the pose in motion at your own pace

Breath
- breath is long and deep
- exhale as you reach forward and inhale as you draw the flowers to your face

Fine points
- eyes are closed if possible
- psychological benefits of this pose are nurturing and healing

Variations
- bend and stretch forward as you reach rather than remaining upright

Inquiry
- "What do you hold most dear?"
- "Who are you, and what do you want?"

Subtle energy visualization (think about, pretend, imagine)
- you are drawing whatever you feel is most precious to you, and as you inhale you are absorbing the essence of it so that it permeates every cell of your body
- fingers are shimmering and sprinkling like sparkles
- drawing to you whatever you hold most dear

Effect
- nourishing, comforting

Benefits
- movement of arms increases lymph flow in axillary area
- rib cage expands for deeper breath capacity
- psychologically soothing

Prone Poses
(on the belly)

View short video clips of the poses being demonstrated online at
www.donnabelk.com/restorativeflow

Wag the Dog's Tail *Ardha Bhujangasana*

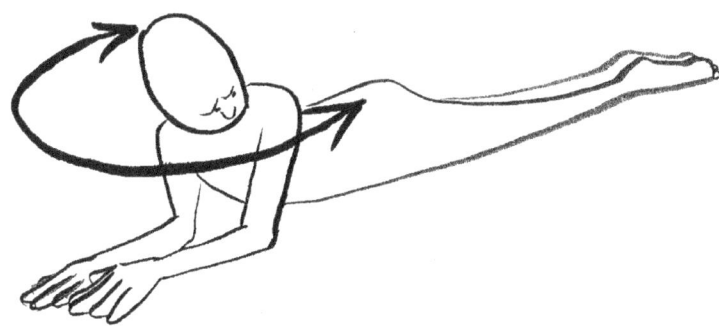

Moving into the pose
- come to a position so you are lying on your belly with your elbows bent and your forearms supporting the weight of your body(like a sphinx)
- lengthen through the spine
- slightly tuck the tailbone
- turn the head to one side to look toward your feet
- come back to center and repeat on other side
- continue the pose in motion, going from side to side

Breath
- breath is easy and natural
- exhale as you turn to the side, and inhale as you come back to center

Fine points
- pace is slow and easy
- shoulders are dropped away from the ears
- palms are flat on the floor
- elbows are underneath shoulders
- hip bones remain on the floor so the sensation is felt more along the sides of the body

Variations
- bend the knees while maintaining the sphinx position
- move the elbows forward if there is discomfort in the back

Inquiry
- "Can you feel the stretch along the side of your body?"

Subtle energy visualization (think about, pretend, imagine)
- follow the line of energy from the shoulder to the tips of your toes

Effect
- harmonizing

Benefits
- lateral stretch for the spine which helps create more space in the space between the vertebrae
- compression and expansion of the ribs

Cobra (3 variations) *Bhujangasana*

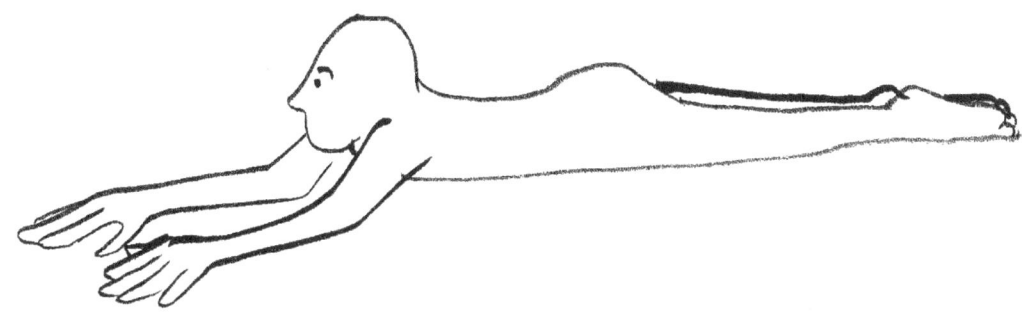

Moving into the pose
- lying on your belly; forehead touching the floor; arms fully extended above your head; palms face the floor
- lengthen through the legs and tuck the tailbone slightly
- on the inhale lift the face to look towards the ceiling
- on the exhale lower the head touching the chin, nose and forehead to the floor
- repeat 3 to 5 times

Breath
- inhale as you look toward the ceiling, exhale as you lower the head
- breath is easy and natural

Fine points
- pace is slow and easy
- shoulders are dropped away from the ears

Variations
- bring the hands in line with the face, elbows rest on the floor tucked in close to the torso
- tuck the hands underneath the shoulders, elbows lifted from the floor and tucked in close to the torso

Inquiry
- "When you are looking toward the ceiling, do you notice the sensation from your belly button all the way up to your chin?"
- "Do you feel a stretch in the back of the neck and shoulders?"

Subtle energy visualization (think about, pretend, imagine)
- the sun is shining down on the spine warming it so it is like an undulating golden river

Effect
- stretching, strengthening

Benefits
- limbers the spine
- stretches the front of the body

Diagonal Stretch

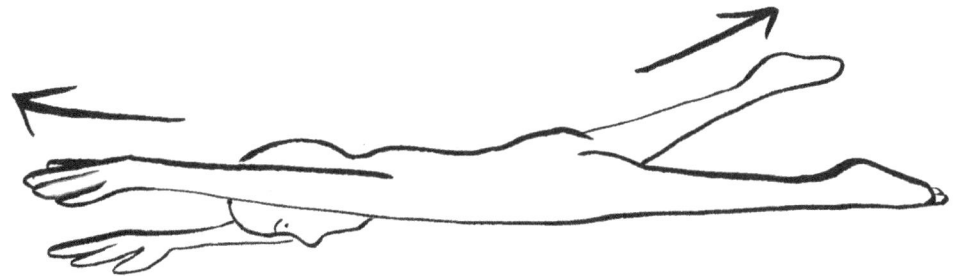

Moving into the pose
- lying on your belly; forehead touching the floor; arms fully extended above your head; palms face the floor
- lengthen through the legs and tuck the tailbone slightly
- lift one arm, stretch and reach toward the wall with the fingertips, hold for 3-5 breaths, then release to the floor
- repeat with the other arm
- repeat with one leg and then the other leg
- repeat with one arm and the opposite leg extended at the same time
- repeat on the other side

Breath
- breath is easy and natural

Fine points
- stretch is gentle and easy
- forehead remains on the floor
- tailbone slightly tucked

Variations
- advanced: lift the head, arms and legs at the same time

Inquiry
- "Can you feel the stretch from your fingertips to your toetips?"

Subtle energy visualization (think about, pretend, imagine)
- trace a light path from toetips to fingertips
- ribbons or streamers of light are anchored in your navel area and then shoot out your fingers and toes

Effect
- harmonizing

Benefits
- limbers the spine
- good for cross-functional brain functioning

Bend the Knees Circling

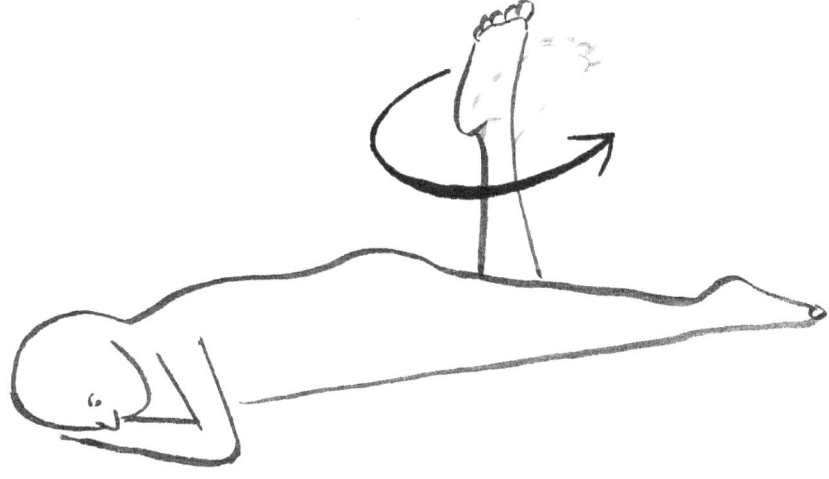

Moving into the pose
- lying on your belly, head turned to one side with the bent arms making a pillow for your head
- bend the knee and circle the ankle; 3 to 5 times in one direction, pause, then reverse directions
- with the knee still bent squeeze the toes together like you were making little fists, then separate the toes as wide as you can; repeat 3 to 5 times
- with the knee still bent circle the entire lower leg, making as big a circle as you can and trying to touch the floor as the leg circles around; 3 to 5 times in one direction, pause, then reverse directions
- pause, turn the head to look the other way, then repeat sequence on the other side with the other leg

Breath
- breath is easy and natural

Fine points
- pace is slow and easy
- eyes resting downward or closed
- soft smile on the lips

Variations
- circle both legs at the same time, in the same direction and then in opposite directions from one another
- cross ankles, separate feel and cross ankles again producing a scissor kick crossing legs back and forth

Inquiry
- "Can you notice how the breath moves in the back of your body?"

Subtle energy visualization (think about, pretend, imagine)
- a loving hand rests on your shoulder or back (or any other area) and the only intent is to soothe you and bring you comfort
- ribbons or streamers of light (anchored in your belly) stream out from your toes as you circle each leg

Effect
- calming, soothing

Benefits
- takes the knee, ankle and toes through their full range of motion
- allows an opportunity to rest on the belly and notice how the breath moves in the back of the body

Turn the Head to One Side

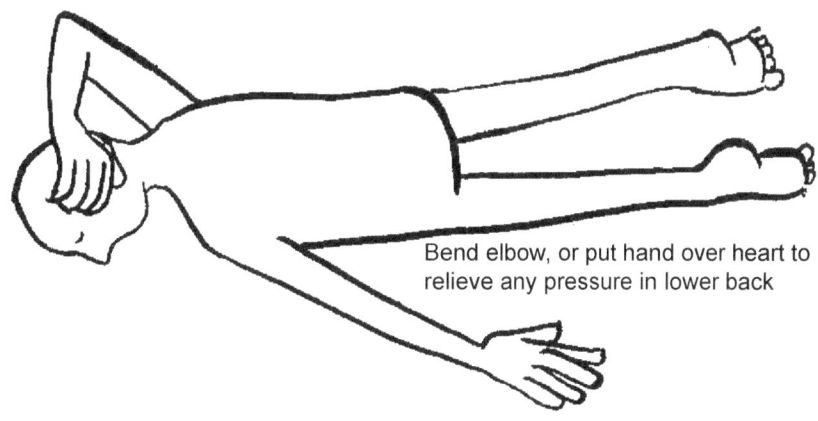

Bend elbow, or put hand over heart to relieve any pressure in lower back

Moving into the pose
- lying on your belly, arms alongside the body, and head resting to one side directly on the floor (not on hands)
- if the head is turned to the right bring the left hand slightly above and behind the right ear
- gently press the back of the head toward the floor creating a stretch in the neck
- hold for 3 to 5 breaths (or even 1-2 minutes), and change to the other side

Breath
- breath is slow and deep

Fine points
- stretch is gentle and easy
- chin is slightly tucked
- knees can be bent if there is too much pressure on the lower back
- eyes resting downward or closed
- the arm that is extended alongside the body can be straight or bent

Variations
- if there is any discomfort in the neck do not use the hand to press the head toward the floor; simply turning the head to the side may be enough stretch for some individuals
- instead of extending the non-working arm alongside the body, roll to one side and place the hand over the heart
- notice
  - how it feels without a hand on the head
  - place hand on head and see how it feels different
  - move hand to different position (on shoulder, for example) and notice how that feels
  - remove hand entirely and notice the difference in sensation

Inquiry
- "In what area of the neck do you feel the most sensation?"
- "Can you feel your belly as it presses against the floor on the inhalation?

Subtle energy visualization (think about, pretend, imagine)
- a loving hand rests on your head, what would this loving being say to you?
- the sun is shining down on the spine warming it

Effect
- soothing, calming, nourishing, focusing

Benefits
- enhances range of motion in the neck area
- calms the nervous system

Side Lying Poses

View short video clips of the poses being demonstrated online at
www.donnabelk.com/restorativeflow

Big Arm Circles

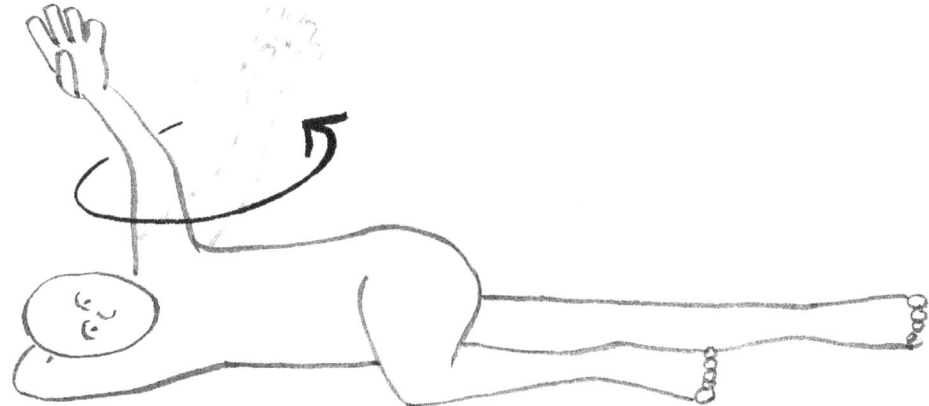

Moving into the pose
- come to a position so you are lying on your side
- one arm is tucked under your head like a pillow (arm can be straight, or elbow bent)
- the bottom leg is straight, upper leg is bent with the knee resting on the floor
- bring the upper arm by the ear, reach and stretch with the fingertips
- begin to circle the arm in as big a circle as you can make, even dragging the fingers along the floor as much as you can in front of you and behind you
- repeat 5-7 times in one direction, pause, then reverse directions

Breath
- breath is easy and natural
- to apply the breath to the movement, exhale as the arm circles forward and inhale as the arm circles behind

Fine points
- pace is slow and easy
- eyes resting downward or closed
- legs are very relaxed
- if someone has discomfort in the shoulder, keep the elbow bent
- bend the elbow if there is any discomfort in the circling arm

Variations
- find a place that feels like a wonderful stretch, pause there for 5-10 breaths
- let the body twist a little as the arm circles behind
- begin by making very tiny circles with the hand pointed to the ceiling, and gradually make the circles larger and larger

Inquiry
- "How deeply in the shoulder girdle can you feel this opening?"

Subtle energy visualization (think about, pretend, imagine)
- with the hand pointing straight up begin to create little spirals and let the spirals continue to get larger and larger
- ribbons of light shoot out the fingertips creating a cocoon of energy around you

Effect
- calming

Benefits
- opens the shoulder area

Elbow to Knee

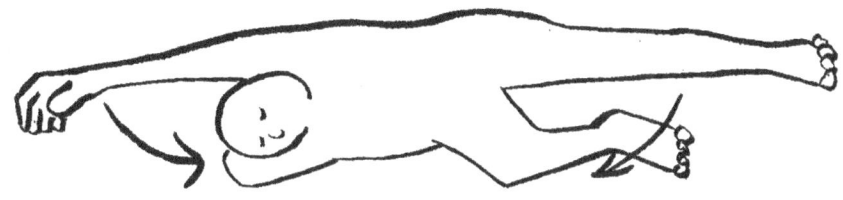

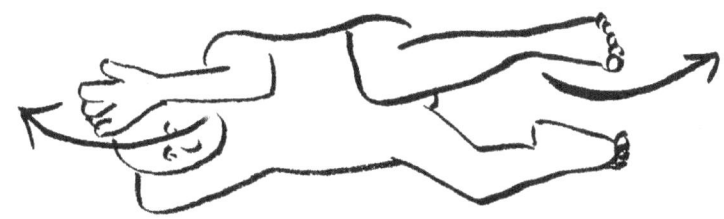

Moving into the pose
- lying on the side of the body
- one arm is tucked under your head like a pillow, or the arm can be straight whatever is most comfortable
- the bottom leg is bent, upper leg is straight
- bring the upper arm by the ear, reach and stretch with the fingertips
- extend the upper leg and reach and stretch with the toetips
- on an exhale bend the elbow and knee so they begin to come together as if to touch each other
- on an inhale extend the arm and leg again reaching and stretching as much as you are able
- continue the pose in motion at your own pace

Breath
- breath is long and deep
- exhale as the elbow and knee come to meet one another, inhale as the leg and arm extend

Fine points
- pace is slow and easy
- eyes resting downward or closed
- as the leg and arm extend, they are parallel to the floor

Variations
- rest the arms and legs to the floor and lie in fetal position while noticing the breath in the back of the body (especially the sacrum)
- arch the back and reach back as far as you can with the arm and leg

Inquiry
- "Can you feel the stretch all along the side of your body?"
- "Where can you not feel the stretch along the side of your body?

Subtle energy visualization (think about, pretend, imagine)
- streamers of light extend from fingers and toes
- drawing in from the universe what you want as you inhale, releasing what no longer serves you as you exhale

Effect
- expansive and contracting

Benefits
- limbers the spine
- lateral stretch for the body

Supine Poses
(on the back)

View short video clips of the poses being demonstrated online at
www.donnabelk.com/restorativeflow

Knees to Chest

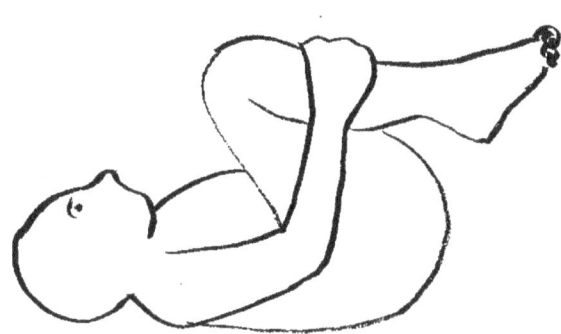

Moving into the pose
- lying on your back draw the knees into the chest
- place the hands on the shins, or on the back of the thighs, or wrap your arms around the legs

Breath
- breath is long and deep

Fine points
- eyes resting downward or closed

Variations
- gently rock from side to side for a gentle back massage
- hold one knee to the chest at a time
- hold one knee to the chest at a time with the other leg extended

Inquiry
- "Notice how the small of the back presses into the floor."

Subtle energy visualization (think about, pretend, imagine)
- trace the energy route along the spine
- trace the energy route in the center of the body from the perineum to the top of the head (thrusting channel or *shushumna*)
- follow or trace the energy route between the eyebrows back to the base of the skull (occipital area)

Effect
- focusing, calming

Benefits
- massages the spine
- massages the internal organs
- this pose is called wind-relieving pose (for obvious reasons)

Sacrum Circles

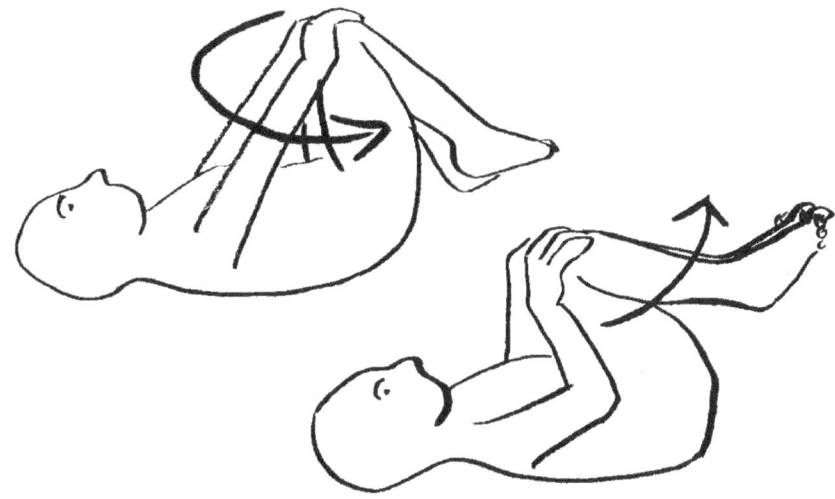

Moving into the pose
- lying on your back draw the knees into the chest
- place the hands on top of the knees
- slowly rotate the knees in a circle trying to feel the sacrum or triangular bone at the base of your spine
- 5-7 times in one direction, pause, then reverse directions

Breath
- breath is easy and natural
- as the knees circle away from the body inhale, and as the knees circle close to the chest exhale

Fine points
- pace is slow and easy
- eyes resting downward or closed

Variations
- rock side to side as you circle the knees

Inquiry
- "Can you trace the outside edges of the sacrum?"
- "Notice the small of the back lifting away from the floor and being pressed into the floor."

Subtle energy visualization (think about, pretend, imagine)
- trace the energy route along the spine
- follow the energy route in the center of the body from the perineum to the top of the head (thrusting channel or shushumna)
- fill the sacrum with light, energy, warmth or sound
- create a circling energy ball in the belly

Effect
- focusing, calming

Benefits
- massages the sacrum area
- massages the internal organs

Knees Bent

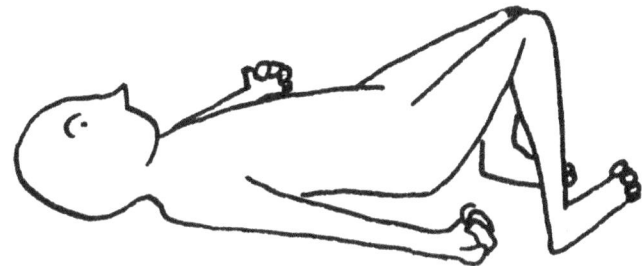

Being on the floor COMFORTABLY can be difficult for some people because of discomfort in the lower back. The Knees Bent posture usually works for everyone and is one of the safest postures for protecting the lower back.

Moving into the pose
- knees are bent with feet separated more than hip-width apart
- bent knees are touching, or resting one against the other (This allows people to stay in the posture without engaging the muscles of the legs and abdomen, which is what makes this pose so relaxing. The body is fully supported, and the lower back is allowed to relax completely.)
- arms are relaxed alongside the body

Fine points
- excellent posture for breathwork

Variations
- this pose is exceptionally soothing and nurturing when people rest their hands on their belly

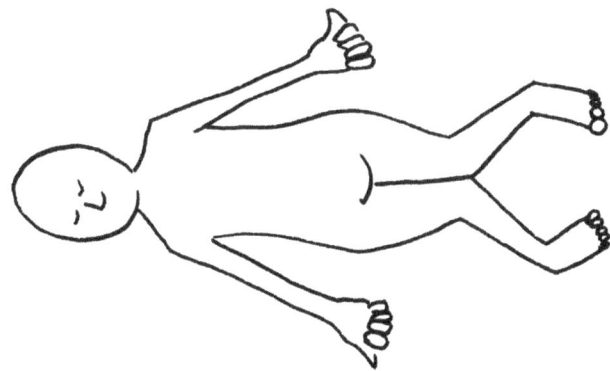

View from above as you would look down on someone in the pose.
Looks funny, feels good!

Inquiry
- Notice the places where the spine touches the floor, and where it does *not* touch the floor
- Can you feel the weight of your belly/

Subtle energy visualization (think about, pretend, imagine)
- create a circling, sparkling energy ball in your belly allow it to expand and contract with each breath
- follow the energy route in the center of the body from the perineum to the top of the head (thrusting channel or *shushumna*)

Effect
- soothing, calming, nourishing

Benefits
- one of the safest positions for the back

Arm Pump

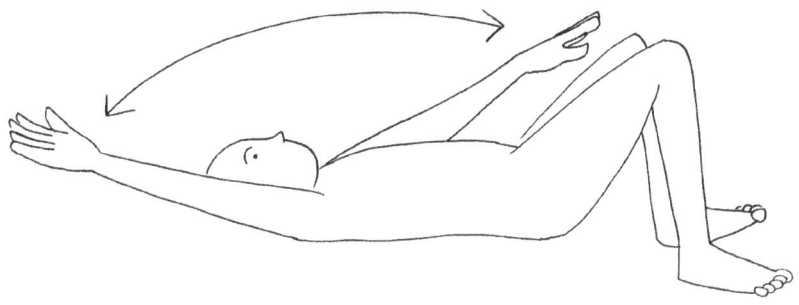

Moving into the pose
- lying on the back, knees are bent, feet flat on the floor
- arms are resting beside the body, palms face the floor
- extend one arm over the head until the back of the hand rests on the floor
- at the same time move both arms so they switch positions (think synchronized swimming)
- repeat in a flowing, back and forth motion

Breath
- breath is long and deep

Fine points
- pace is slow and easy
- press the small of the back into the floor
- eyes resting downward or closed
- chin is slightly tucked

Variations
- try to coordinate the movement so that the hands touch the floor at the same time

Inquiry
- "Can you feel the stretch along the side of your body?"
- "Notice as the small of the back presses into the floor."

Subtle energy visualization (think about, pretend, imagine)
- ribbons of light or energy extend from the fingers creating undulating lines of color and shapes

Effect
- harmonizing, soothing, calming

Benefits
- massages the axillary area helping distribute lymph throughout the system
- opens the shoulders
- improves right- and left-side coordination

Easy Bridge *Setubandhasana*

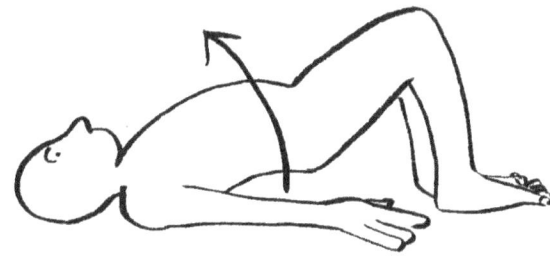

Moving into the pose
- lying on the back with the knees bent and the feet flat on the floor near the buttocks
- align the knees so that they are over the ankles, and about hip-width apart
- press the lower back into the floor and begin to press with the feet to lift the hips from the floor
- lift the hips as high off the floor as you are able, weight is on shoulders and feet
- when you have raised as high as you are able then slowly lower the hips to the floor one vertebrae at a time
- continue the pose in motion at your own pace

Breath
- breath is long and deep
- inhale as the hips lift from the floor, exhale as the hips return to the floor

Fine points
- pace is slow and easy
- eyes resting downward or closed
- arms resting alongside the body
- chin slightly tucked
- shoulders away from the ears

Variations
- when the hips are lifted clasp the hands underneath the body and roll the shoulders back
- hold while in a raised position for 3-5 breaths

Inquiry
- "Can you feel each vertebrae individually, or do they seem to move in sections?"

Subtle energy visualization (think about, pretend, imagine)
- ground into the earth with the hands and activate the spinal energy as the hips lift from the floor
- the spine is like a pearl necklace lying on a dresser, lift the necklace from the dresser one pearl at a time, and as you lift your hips do so one vertebrae at a time

Effect
- soothing, calming, focusing

Benefits
- massages the spine
- opens the chest, hips and front of thighs

Supine Hip Opener

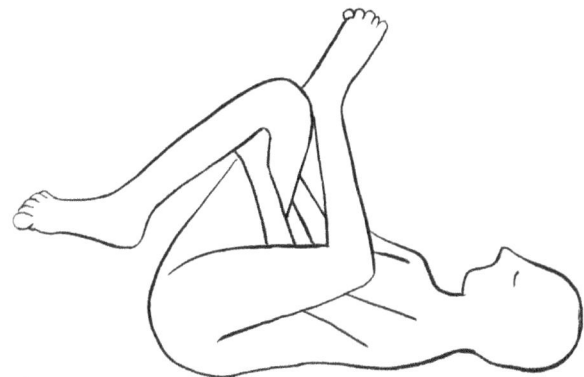

Moving into the pose
- lying on the back with the knees bent and the feet flat on the floor
- place the foot of one leg on the thigh (above the knee) of the other, pressing the bent knee away from the torso
- hold for 1-2 minutes
- release the legs and return to center
- reverse the position of the legs and repeat on other side

Breath
- breath is easy and natural

Fine points
- shoulders are relaxed back
- stretch is easy and gentle
- eyes resting downward or closed

Variations
- leave foot on floor rather than lifting it
- draw the foot of the bent knee closer to the groin for more intensity
- rock gently from side to side for a spinal massage

Inquiry
- "Can you feel the stretch in your hip or bottom?

Subtle energy visualization (think about, pretend, imagine)
- follow the energy route in the center of the body from the perineum to the top of the head (thrusting channel or shushumna)

Effect
- calming, focusing

Benefits
- opens the hips
- massages the sacrum

Pelvic Tilt

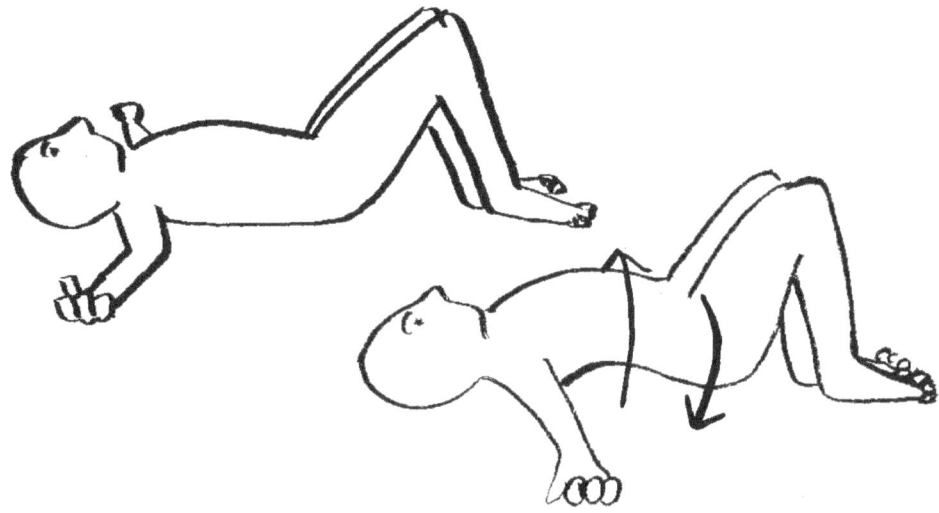

Moving into the pose
- lying on the back with the knees bent and the feet flat on the floor
- press the lower back into the floor trying to flatten the spine
- release
- continue the pose in motion at your own pace

Breath
- breath is easy and natural
- to apply the breath to the movement, exhale as you press the small of the back into the floor, inhale as you release

Fine points
- pace is slow and easy
- eyes resting downward or closed

Variations
- hold for 2-5 breaths when the small of the back is pressing into the floor (but remember to breathe!)
- move arms above the head during inhale, lower to rest beside the hips during exhale
- Rolling Hip Stretch: roll onto outside edges of feet, inhale/exhale and roll knees to the other side, repeat back and forth (widen the feet for more stretch)

Inquiry
- "Can you feel the belly button draw towards the spine as you flatten the back into the floor?"

Subtle energy visualization (think about, pretend, imagine)
- as the small of the back presses into the floor, draw energy or light into the belly; as the pelvis tilts in the opposite direction the energy flows upward in a fountain of light, or sound

Effect
- soothing, focusing

Benefits
- limbers the spine
- brings focus into the lower pelvic area

Spinal Twist *Jathara Parivartanasana*

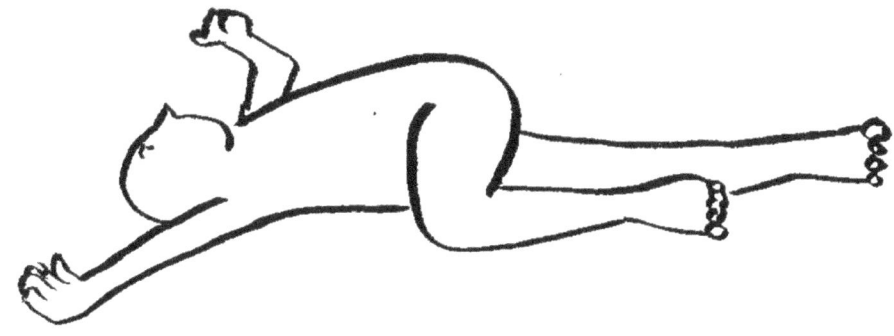

Moving into the pose
- lying on the back with the knees bent and the feet flat on the floor
- arms are in line with the shoulders
- allow the knees to drop toward the floor on one side as the head turns to the other side
- return to center, and repeat on the other side
- continue the pose in motion at your own pace

Breath
- breath is easy and natural
- exhale as the knees travel toward the floor, inhale as the knees return to center

Fine points
- pace is slow and easy
- shoulders remain on the floor
- arms are no higher than the shoulders
- eyes resting downward or closed
- chin is slightly tucked
- palms can be facing the ceiling or pressed to the floor

Variations
- lift the feet slightly from the floor
- hold the pose on one side for 2-5 breaths, or whatever feels delightful
- head in one of three positions
  1. same direction as the knees
  2. neutral
  3. opposite direction as the knees
- tender knees may need blanket to rest on

Inquiry
- "Where do you feel the stretch?"
- "Think of your internal organs are they're being pressed and massaged."

Subtle energy visualization (think about, pretend, imagine)
- energy spirals from the sacrum area all the way up the body massaging and surrounding the internal organs with light and sound

Effect
- soothing, calming, nourishing

Benefits
- limbers the spine
- massages the internal organs

Circle between the Shoulders

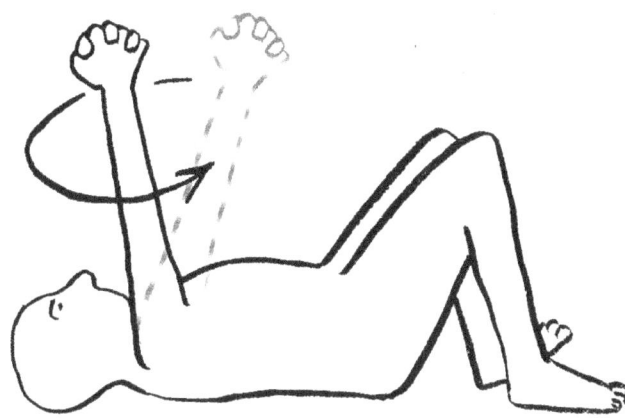

Moving into the pose
- lying on the back with the knees bent and the feet flat on the floor
- clasp hands together and reach the hands toward the ceiling lifting the shoulders from the floor (must lift shoulders from the floor in order to isolate the subtly of this movement)
- circle the clasped hands like you're stirring a pot or drawing a circle on the ceiling
- try to isolate the movement so you feel it between the shoulder blades
- circle 5-7 times, pause, then reverse directions

Breath
- breath is long and deep

Fine points
- pace is slow and easy
- eyes resting downward or closed

Variations
- move the arms like you were chopping wood instead of circling the hands, raising them overhead and then lowering them to the belly
- draw a figure 8 with the hands
- move knees back and forth slightly as the hands move

Inquiry
- "Can you feel the stretch in the hollow between the shoulder blades?"

Subtle energy visualization (think about, pretend, imagine)
- create a circling, sparkling energy ball in the back of your body between your shoulder blades
- holding an imaginary candle in your hands, create big arcs of light as the hands pump up and down

Effect
- soothing, calming

Benefits
- massages the area between the shoulder blades which is a difficult area to stimulate

Lying Tree Pose

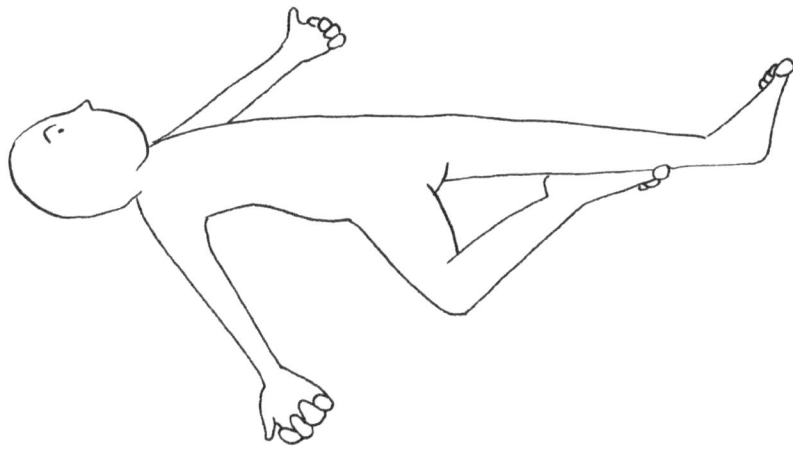

Moving into the pose
- lying on the back with the knees bent and the feet flat on the floor
- extend one leg so it is resting straight along the floor
- allow the other knee to open and fall toward the floor
- hold for 2-5 minutes
- come back to center, reverse the position of the legs and repeat on other side

Breath
- breath is long and deep

Fine points
- arms resting comfortably alongside the body
- stretch is easy and gentle
- eyes resting downward or closed

Variations
- place the foot on top of the thigh for a more intense stretch, being careful not to bend at the ankle
- rest the bent knee on a blanket, or place a fist under the upper thigh to support the bent knee
- arms can be up resting above the head rather than beside the body

Inquiry
- "Can you feel the stretch along the inner thigh?"
- "How does your lower back feel?" [Note: if there is discomfort in the lower back then the straight leg can bend to take the pressure off the lower back.]

Subtle energy visualization (think about, pretend, imagine)
- follow the energy route in the center of the body from the perineum to the top of the head (thrusting channel or *shushumna*)
- expand the heart to fill the room with light, energy or sound

Effect
- soothing, calming, nourishing

Benefits
- opens the hips and chest
- stretch for the inner thighs
- pelvis benefits from a steady supply of blood

Lying Cobbler's Pose (Bound Angle)

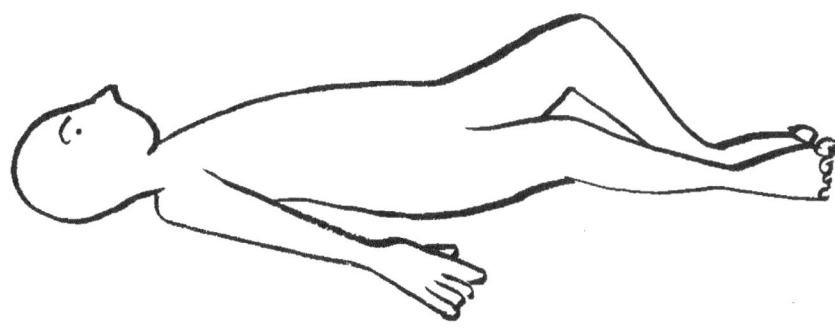

Moving into the pose
- lying on the back with the knees bent and the feet flat on the floor
- allow the knees to open and fall toward the floor so the soles of the feet face one another (experiment to find the best heel/groin distance for your body by moving the feet closer or further away)
- hold for 2-5 minutes

Breath
- breath is long and deep

Fine points
- arms resting comfortably alongside the body
- stretch is gentle and easy
- eyes resting downward or closed
- if there is too much pressure on the inner thighs, or discomfort in the lower back have students move their feet away from their body so there is less bend in the knees

Variations
- for a more intense stretch draw the feet closer to the groin
- to support the knees, roll to one side and place fist under buttock, then roll to other side and place fist under buttock
- lift the feet from the floor and hold the knees

Inquiry
- "Can you feel the stretch along the inner thigh?"
- "How does your lower back feel?"
- "Can you surrender any holding in the belly or hips to the gentle force of gravity?"

Subtle energy visualization (think about, pretend, imagine)
- follow the energy route in the center of the body from the perineum to the top of the head (thrusting channel or shushumna)
- expand the heart to fill the room with light, energy or sound

Effect
- soothing, calming, nourishing

Benefits
- opens the hips and chest
- stretch for the inner thighs
- pelvis benefits from a steady supply of blood

Savasana

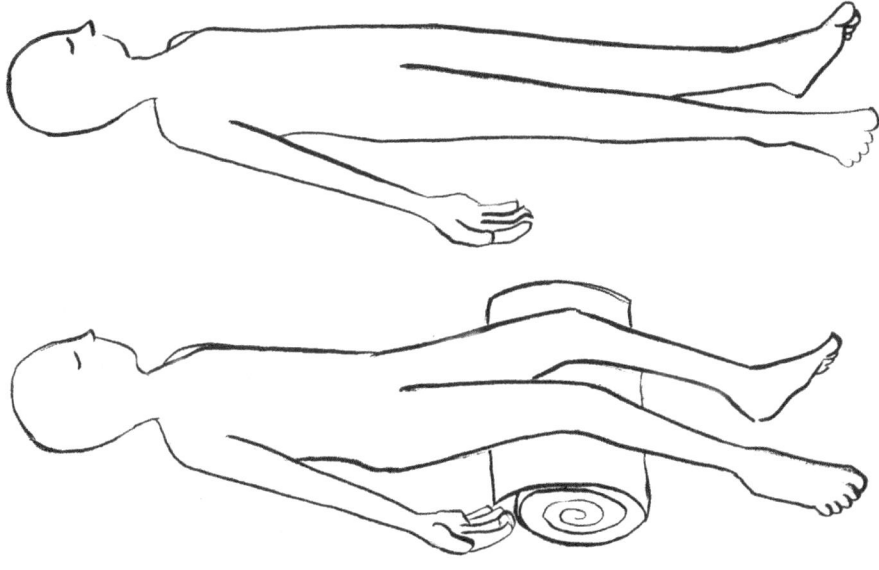

Moving into the pose
- lying on the back with the knees bent and feet flat on the floor
- place a blanket under the knees, if needed, and slide one leg forward until it is straight and then the other

Breath
- breath is long and deep

Fine points
- alignment of body seems symmetrical
- head in line with the spine (not tilted to one side)
- shoulders away from the ears
- neck elongated (chin not jutting up toward the ceiling)
- notice any tension in student's face (frowning, furrowing the brow, jaw clenched)
- notice any tension in student's hands (clenching into fists)
- belly rises and falls as student is breathing and the breath is long and deep

Variations
- lie on side or belly
- move or adjust at any time to make yourself be more comfortable

Inquiry
- "Can you feel your heart beat?"

Subtle energy visualization (think about, pretend, imagine)
- expand the heart to fill the room with light, energy or sound

Effect
- soothing, calming, nourishing, reflective

Benefits
- lowers blood pressure

Poses Using the Wall

Legs Up the Wall *Viparita Karani*

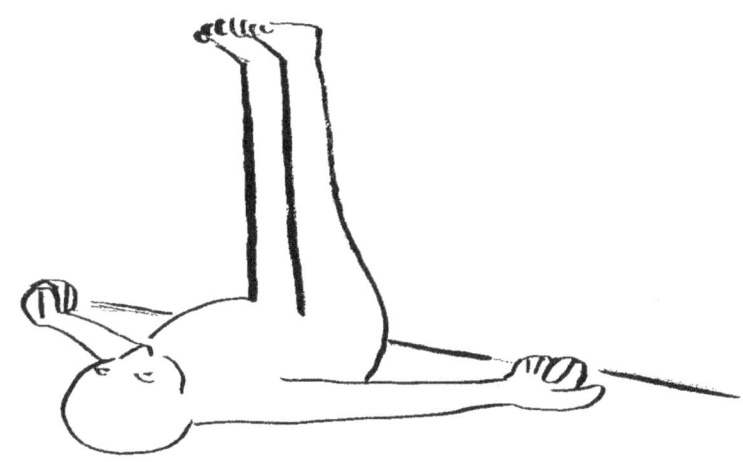

Moving into the pose
- from all fours position, scoot close to the wall so one hip is touching the wall
- lay down on the floor from that position (Hint: it is v-e-r-y important that the torso be perpendicular to the wall)
- roll over onto the back and bring the legs up the wall

Breath
- breath is long and deep

Fine points
- lengthen through the back of the neck and head so the chin is not jutting toward the ceiling
- eyes resting downward or closed
- swallow and relax the throat
- people with high blood pressure should not stay in this long

Variations
- practice this with a lift underneath the hips, especially if the hamstrings are tight
- some students may feel more comfortable with a lift underneath the head
- hands above the head resting on the floor
- hands resting on the belly
- flex the toes back and forth

Inquiry
- "Imagine the blood leaving the legs and pooling in the lower belly before making its way into the heart."
- "Can you notice the rise and fall of your belly as you inhale and exhale?"

Subtle energy visualization (think about, pretend, imagine)
- draw in energy from the bottoms of the feet bringing it all the way up and out the top of the head

Effect
- soothing, calming, nourishing

Benefits
- lowers blood pressure

Legs in "V"

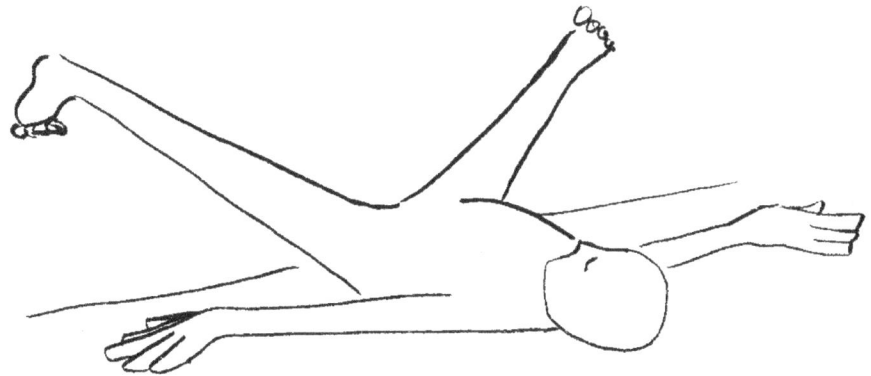

Moving into the pose
- from legs against the wall position, allow the legs to separate and drop toward the floor
- swallow and relax the throat

Breath
- breath is easy and natural

Fine points
- for less intensity bring the legs closer together
- lengthen through the back of the neck and head so the chin is not jutting toward the ceiling
- stretch is gentle and easy
- eyes are closed or resting downward
- swallow and relax the throat
- rest tongue in the floor of the mouth

Variations
- use the hands to support the thighs if the stretch is too intense, or use the hands to press the legs apart if more intensity is wanted

Inquiry
- "Where do you feel the most intense stretch?"

Subtle energy visualization (think about, pretend, imagine)
- draw in energy from the bottoms of the feet bringing it all the way up and pooling in the belly creating a warm, spiraling, sparkling energy ball

Effect
- soothing, calming, nourishing

Benefits
- lowers blood pressure
- stretch for inner thighs

Easy Bridge

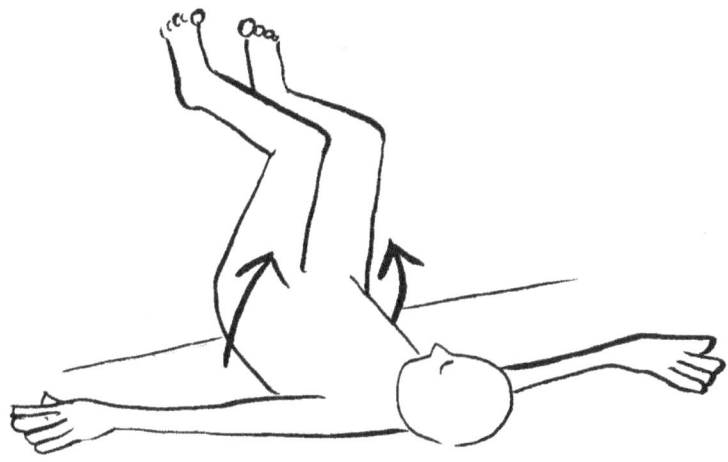

Moving into the pose
- from chair pose against the wall position, the knees are bent and the feet are flat on the wall
- make sure you can see your feet beyond your knees so they are higher toward the ceiling than the knees
- press against the wall and begin to lift the hips from the floor
- when you've gone as high as is comfortable roll back down to the floor a vertebrae at a time
- continue the pose in motion, rolling up and coming down

Breath
- breath is easy and natural

Fine points
- pace is slow and easy
- adjust the feet on the wall away from the hips or toward the hips to be more comfortable
- keep the head in one position, not turning from side to side
- eyes are closed or resting downward
- if there are neck concerns it helps to have a lift under the head or neck

Variations
- when student is in the uppermost position place the hands under the hips to hold them and step one foot away from the wall and then the other into Candle (beginning shoulderstand) position

Inquiry
- "Is it easier for your feet to be further away from your hips, or nearer your hips?"
- "Can you feel the individual vertebrae in the spine as you roll up and down?"

Subtle energy visualization (think about, pretend, imagine)
- trace energy or light up and down the spine

Effect
- soothing, calming

Benefits
- lowers blood pressure
- limbers the spine

Hip Opener

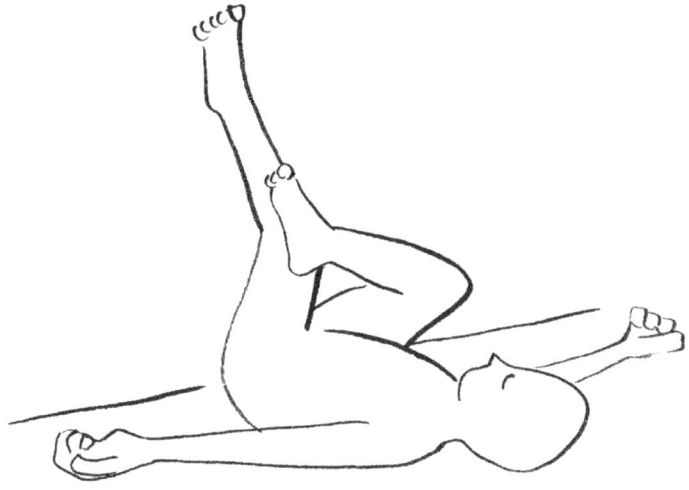

Moving into the pose
- begin with legs straight up the wall; place one ankle so it rests on the thigh of the other leg (Example: allow your right ankle to rest just above your left knee on the thigh)
- begin to bend the straight leg until you feel a comfortable stretch in the opposite hip (Example: bend the left leg and feel a stretch in the right hip)

Breath
- breath is long and deep

Fine points
- move the foot against the wall closer to the hips or further away to intensify the stretch in the hips
- lengthen through the back of the neck and head so the chin is not jutting toward the ceiling
- stretch is gentle and easy
- eyes are closed or resting downward

Variations
- slide ankle up and down the thigh to adjust intensity of stretch
- press one hand against the bent knee toward the wall if a more intense stretch is desired

Inquiry
- "Where do you feel the intensity of the stretch?"
- "Can you feel into the hip joint? Allow it to soften and open."

Subtle energy visualization (think about, pretend, imagine)
- draw in energy from the bottom of the foot of the straight leg bringing it all the way into the belly, then send it out the bottom of the foot again

Effect
- soothing, calming, nourishing

Benefits
- lowers blood pressure
- opens the hip

Cobbler's Pose

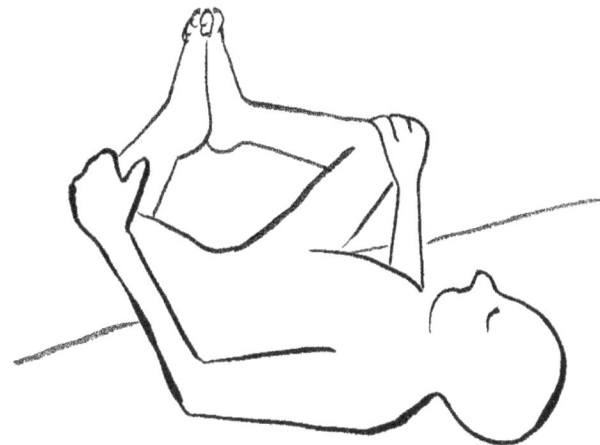

Moving into the pose
- from legs up the wall position, bend both legs drawing the feet close to the groin

Breath
- breath is easy and natural

Fine points
- lengthen through the back of the neck and head so the chin is not jutting toward the ceiling
- stretch is gentle and easy
- eyes are closed or resting downward

Variations
- to intensify the stretch draw the feet closer to the groin
- keep one leg straight as the other leg is bent
- use the hands to press against the knees toward the wall to create more intensity

Inquiry
- "Where do you feel the most intensity?"
- "Can you press the small of the back toward the floor? What happens to the spine when you do that?

Subtle energy visualization (think about, pretend, imagine)
- lead energy, light or sound up and down the spin

Effect
- soothing, calming

Benefits
- lowers blood pressure
- limbers the inner thigh muscles

Knees to Chest

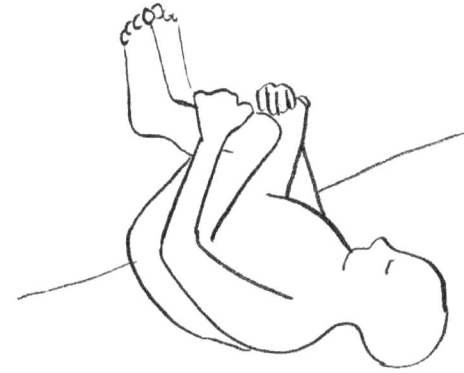

Moving into the pose
- from legs up the wall position, draw the knees in to the chest

Breath
- breath is easy and natural

Fine points
- lengthen through the back of the neck and head so the chin is not jutting toward the ceiling (tuck the chin and grow the neck long)
- stretch is gentle and easy
- eyes are closed or resting downward

Variations
- from this position you can go into a spinal twist against the wall
- lift the head drawing the chin in toward the chest
- gently rock from side to side for a gentle back massage
- hold one knee to the chest at a time with the other leg extended along the wall

Inquiry
- "Does this feel comforting to your body?"

Subtle energy visualization (think about, pretend, imagine)
- create a ball of energy, light, warmth or sound in the belly and circle the ball

Effect
- soothing, calming, nourishing

Benefits
- lowers blood pressure
- massages the internal organs

Chest Expander or Heart Opening Pose
(Can be used with one or two blankets)

Step 1 (below): Fold one blanket into a zigzag or accordion fold.

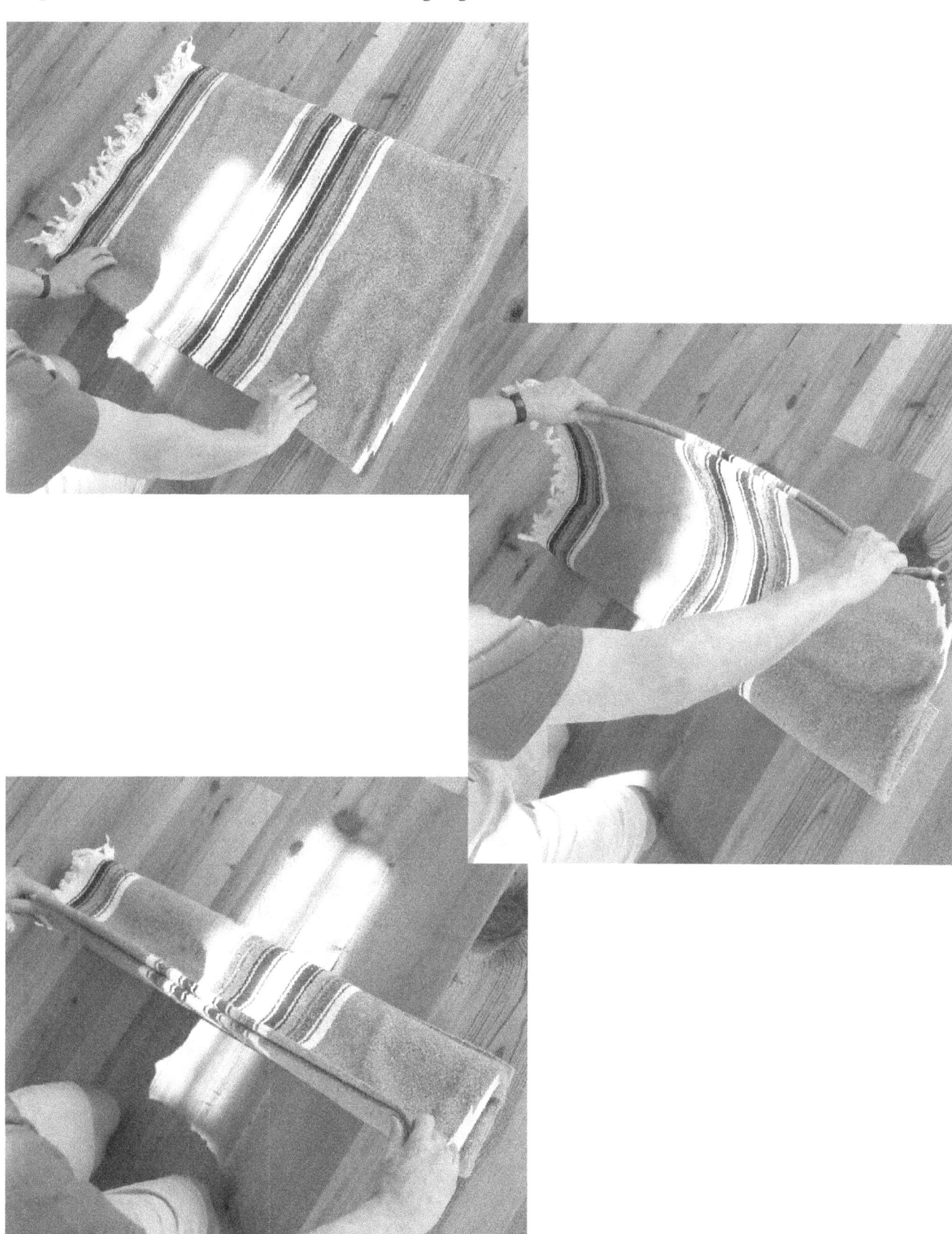

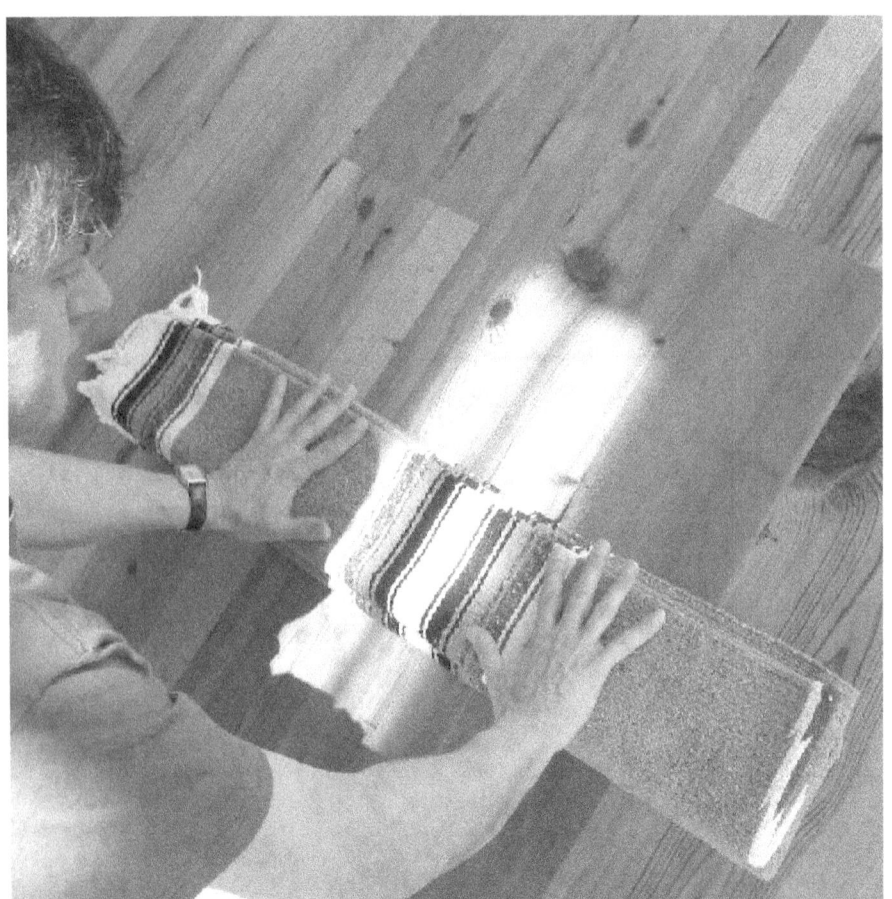

Step 2 (left): Smooth out the blanket(s) making sure the lift is wrinkle free.

Step 3 (right):
Fold a second blanket and place it on top of the first blanket. This is optional. If you prefer a lower lift then use ony one blanket.

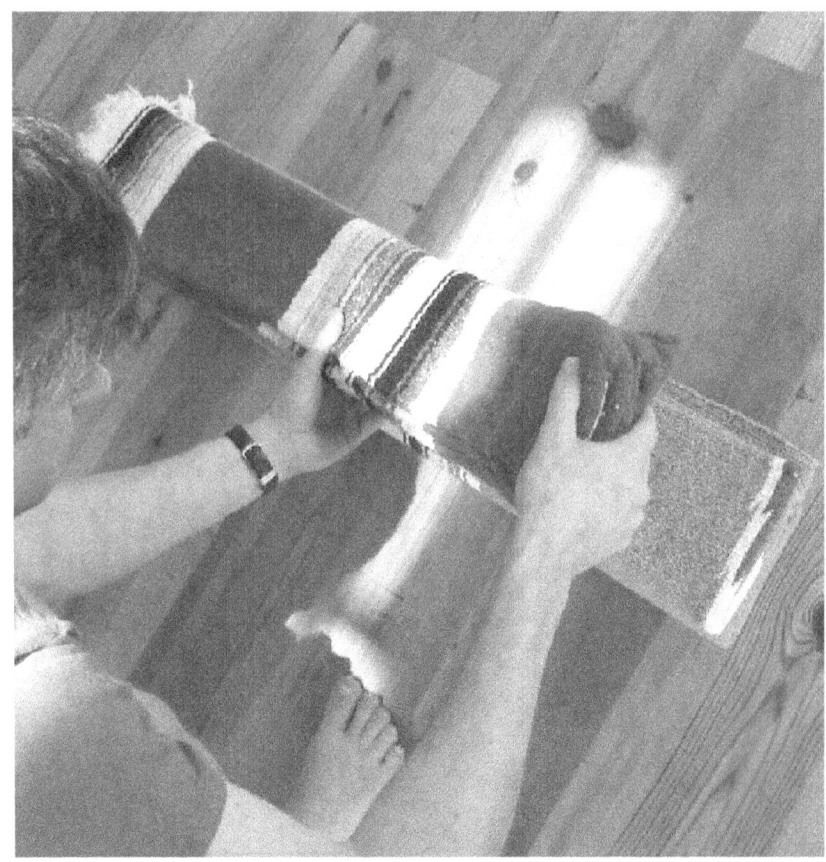

Model is Charles Macinerney, yoga teacher, Austin, Texas

Step 4 (below): Position blanket(s) at the base of the spine without sitting on it

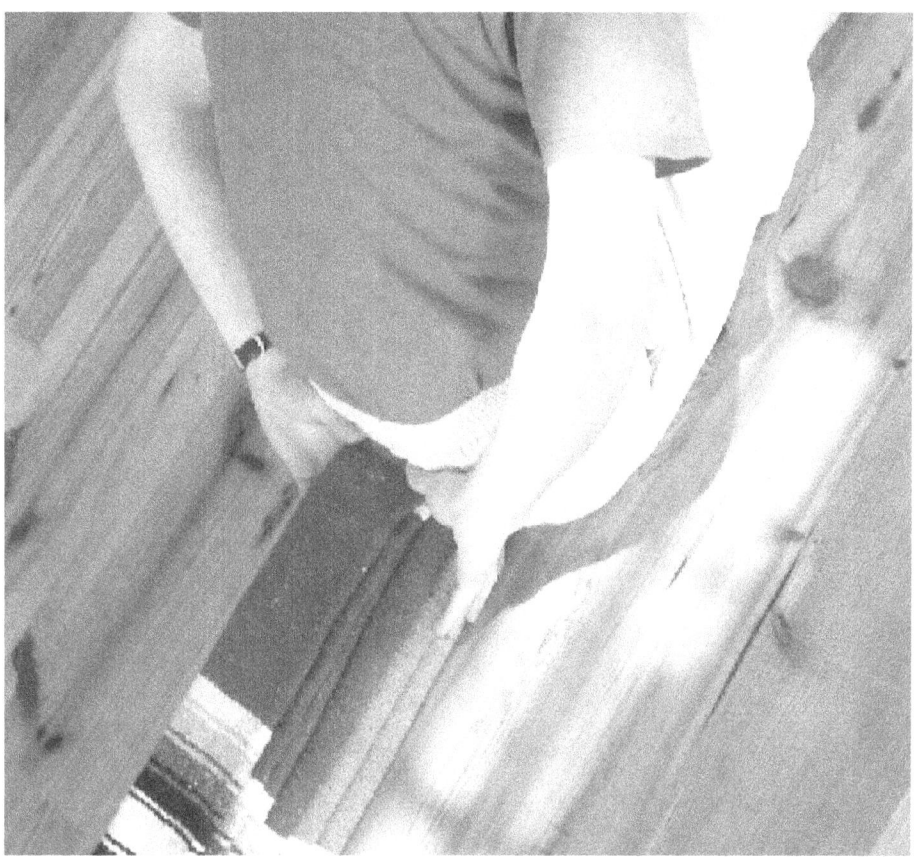

Step 5 (below): Relax back onto the blankets. Tuck the end of the top blanket under the neck for additional comfort and support. If there is any discomfort in the lower back bend the knees. Enjoy!!

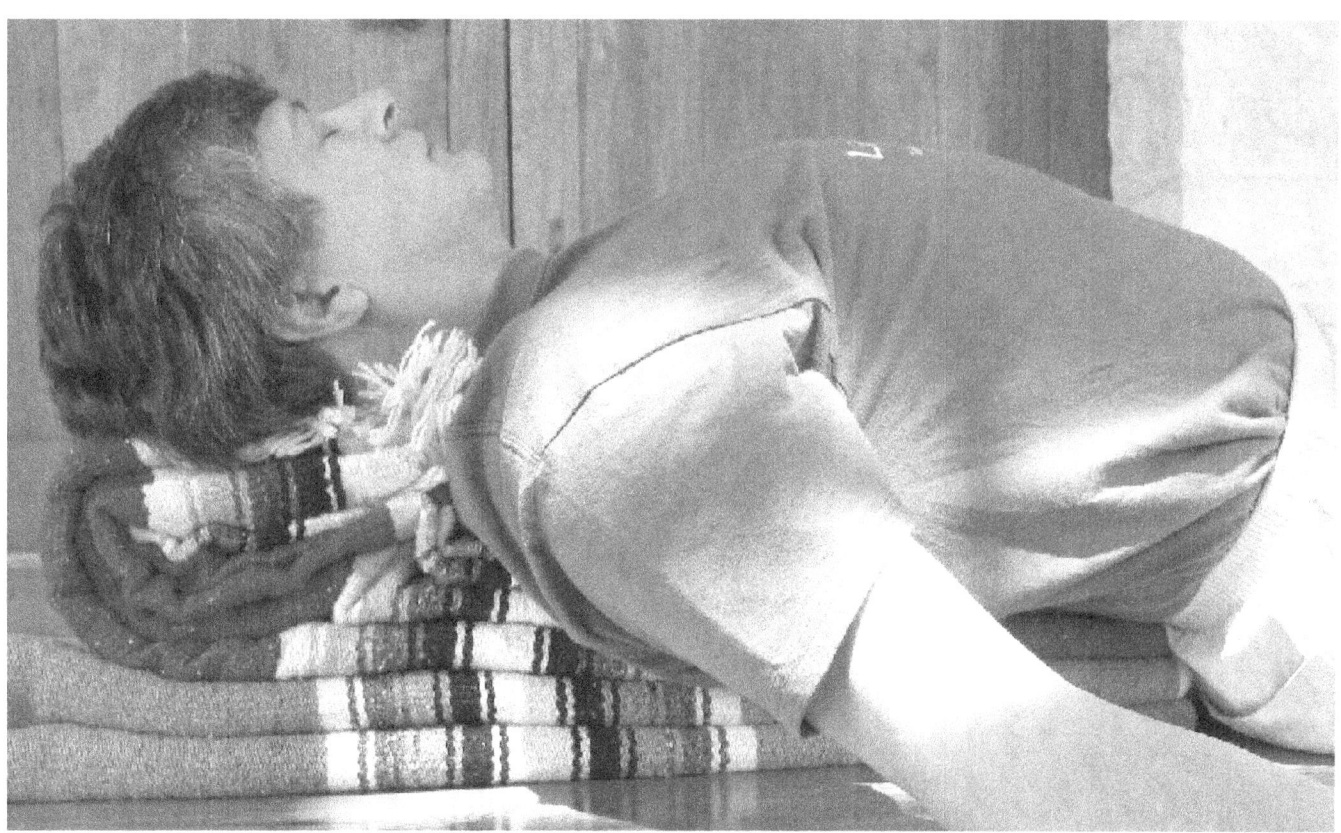

Poses organized by position: all fours, seated, prone, side-lying, supine, standing

Poses on All Fours

Cat & Cow

Thread the Needle

Child's Pose (cradling the face)

Moving Child's Pose

Seated Poses

Circle all the Joints
- toes
- ankles
- top of foot
- knees
- hips
- wrists
- elbows
- shoulders
- neck
- jaw

Torso Circles

Seated Triangle

Seated Cobra

Easy Seated Forward Bend

Easy Seated Twist

Stir the Pot

Moving Seated Forward Bend

Animal Stretch

Gathering Breath

Prone Poses

Wag the Dog's Tail

Cobra (3 variations)

Diagonal Stretch

Bend the Knees Circling

Turn the Head to One Side

Side Lying Poses

Big Arm Circles

Elbow to Knee

Supine Poses

Knees to Chest

Sacrum Circles

Pelvic Tilt

Easy Bridge

Supine Hip Opener

Circle Between Shoulders

Spinal Twist

Lying Tree Pose

Lying Cobbler's Pose

Savasana

Standing Poses

Circle all the Joints

- toes
- ankles
- top of foot
- knees
- hips
- wrists
- elbows
- shoulders
- neck
- jaw

Forward and Backbending

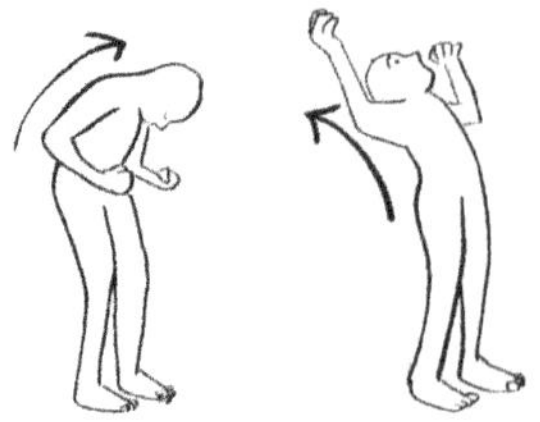

Flying Tadasana

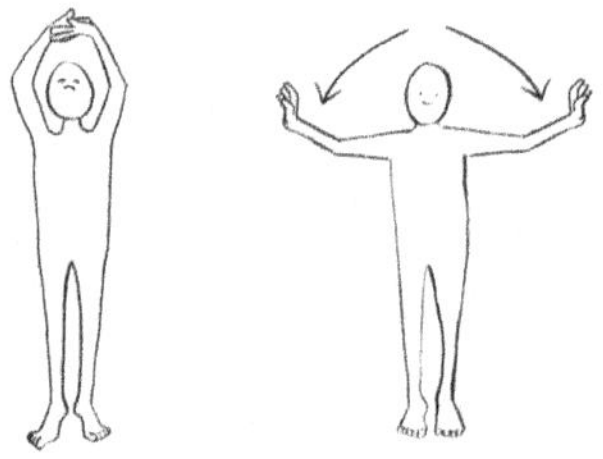

Lift the Arms and Toes

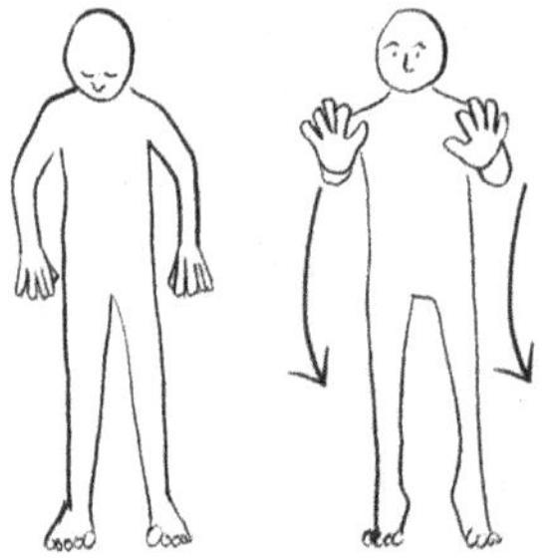

Easy Triangle

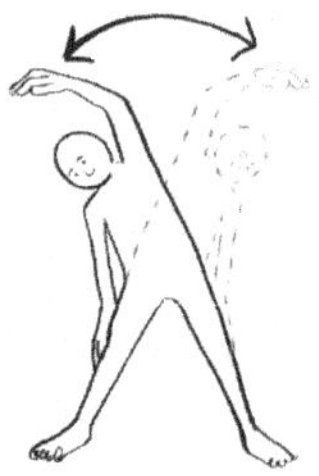

Horse Stance

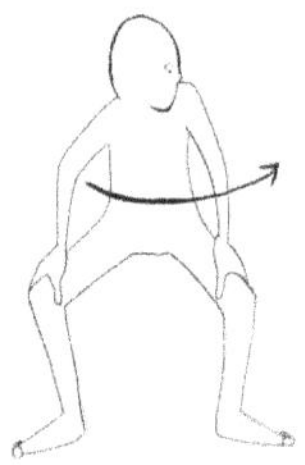

Windmill

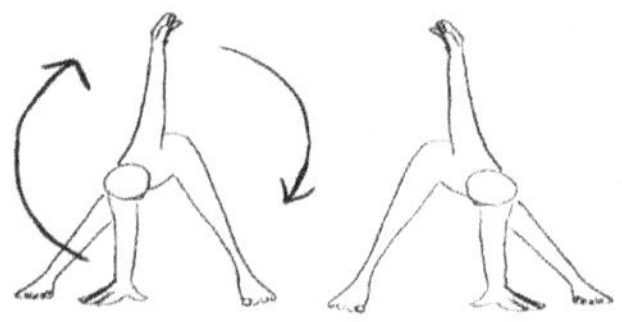

Poses Using the Wall

Legs Up the Wall

Easy Bridge

Legs in "V"

Hip Opener

Cobbler's Pose

Knees to Chest

Sample Classes

Chair Class

Although the poses pictured here are NOT in a chair, the poses themselves can all be done in a chair with the person sitting toward the edge of the seat.

Circle all the Joints	Forward and Backbending of the Spine
• toes • wrists • ankles • elbows • top of foot • shoulders • knees • neck • hips • jaw	
Flying Tadasana	**Horse stance** (focus on shoulders)
Moving Triangle	**Big Arm Circles**

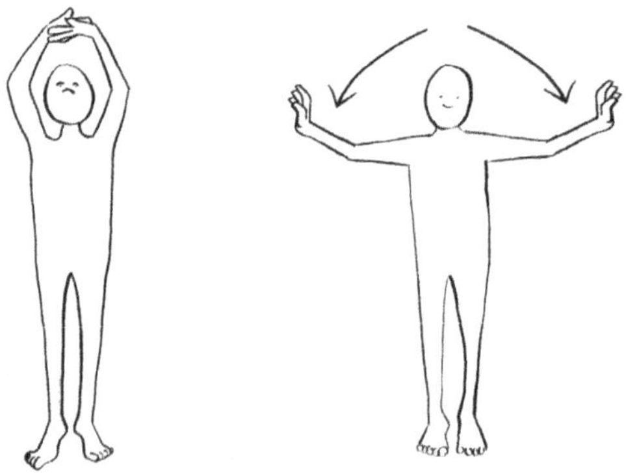

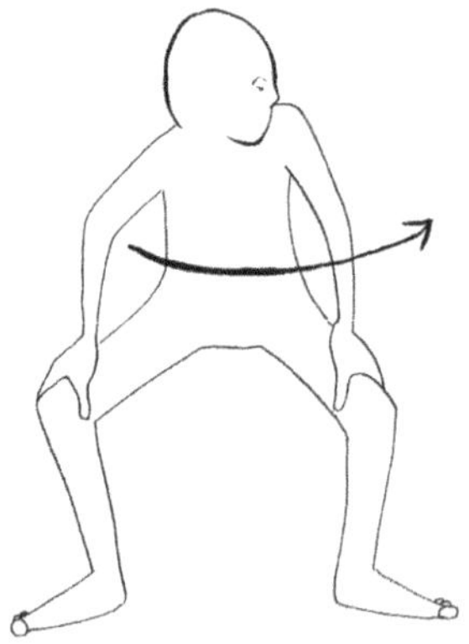

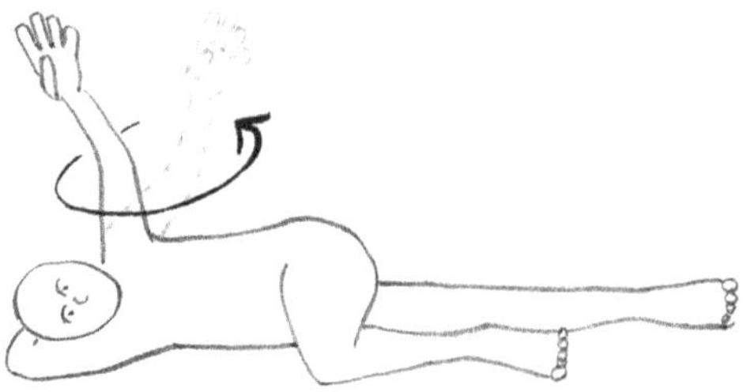

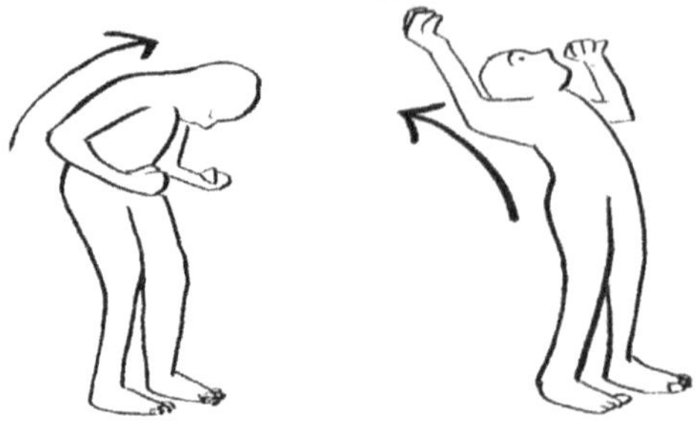

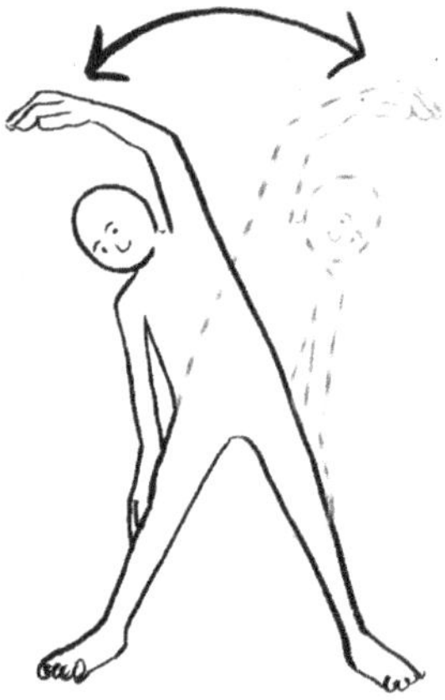

General Class 1: Standing, All Fours, Prone, Supine

Circle all the Joints

- toes
- ankles
- top of foot
- knees
- hips
- wrists
- elbows
- shoulders
- neck
- jaw

Forward and Backbending of the Spine

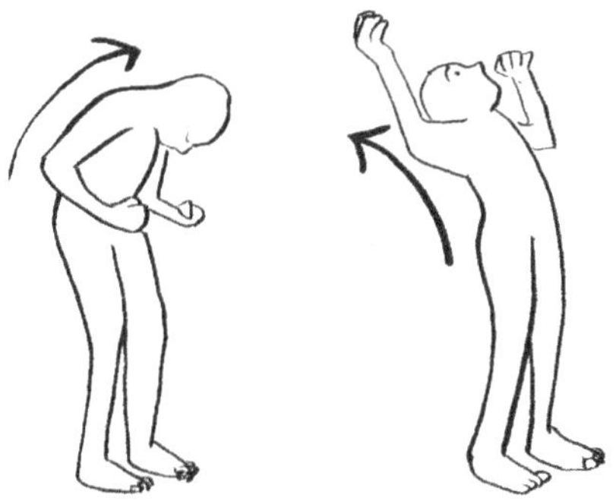

Flying Tadasana

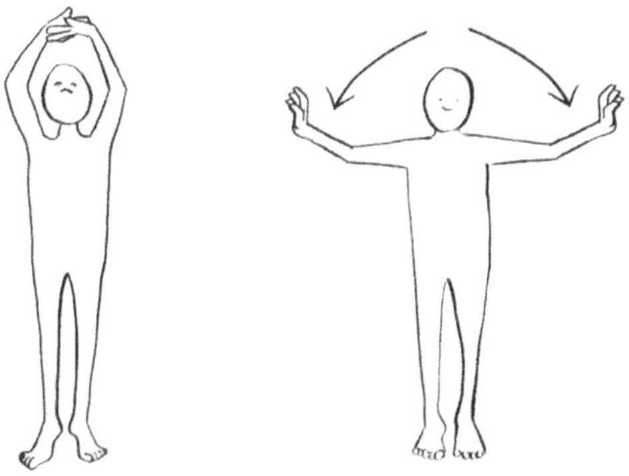

Easy Triangle

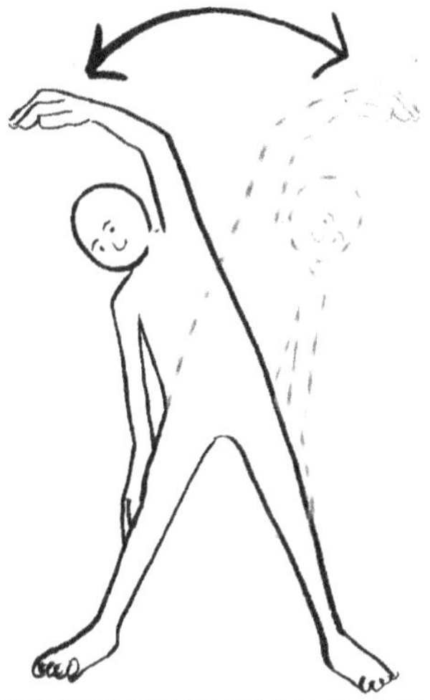

Lift the Arms and Lift the Toes

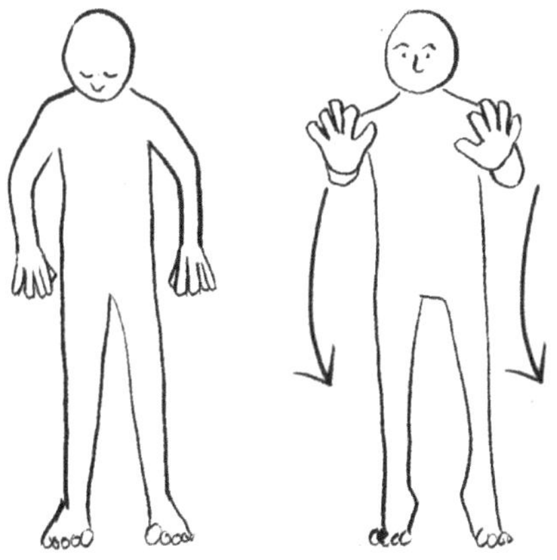

Horse stance

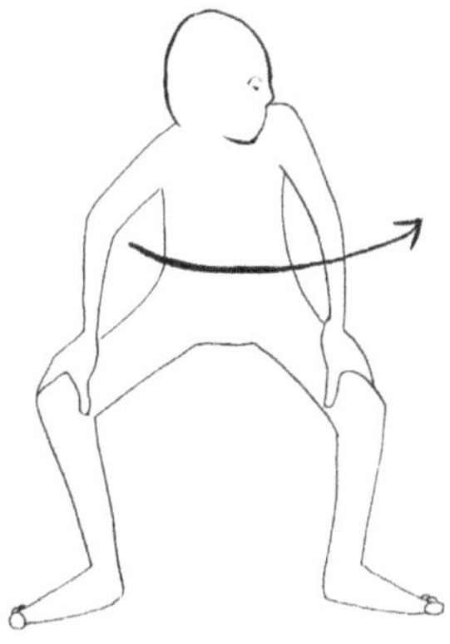

Windmill	Cat & Cow (Cat stretch)
Child's Pose (cradling the face OR Inner Thigh Stretch)	**Moving Child's Pose**
Thread the Needle	**Wag the Dog's Tail**
Diagonal Stretch	**Cobra** (3 of them)

Bend the Knees Circling	**Turn the Head to One Side**
Knees to Chest	**Supine Hip Opener**
Spinal Twist	**Savasana**

General Class 2: Seated, Prone, Supine, page 1

Circle all the Joints

- toes
- ankles
- top of foot
- knees
- hips
- wrists
- elbows
- shoulders
- neck
- jaw

Torso Circles

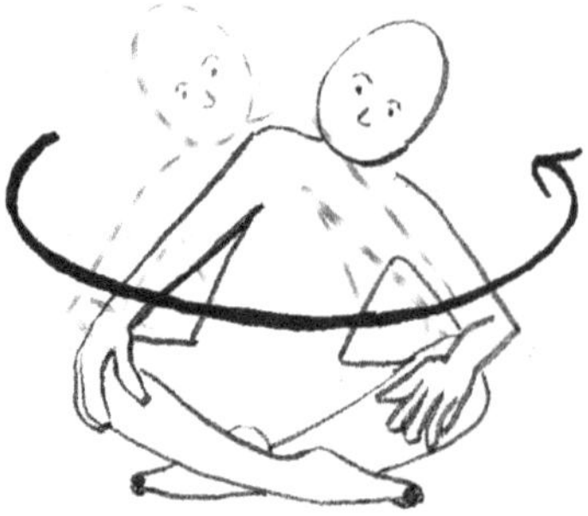

Seated Triangle

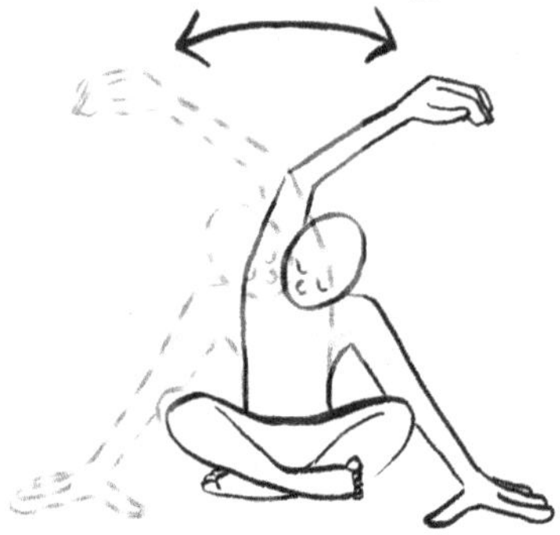

Easy Seated Twist

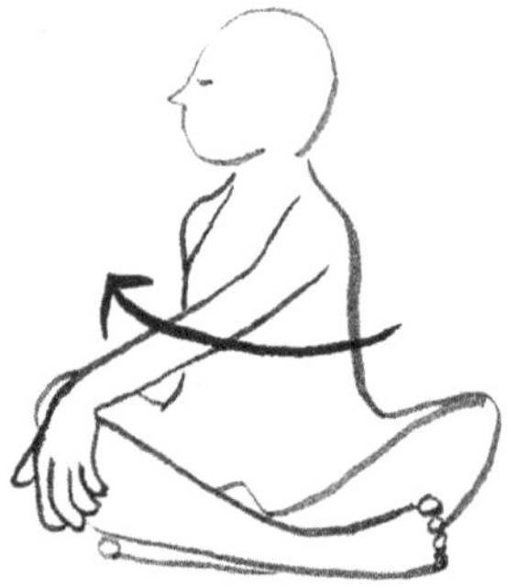

Animal Stretch

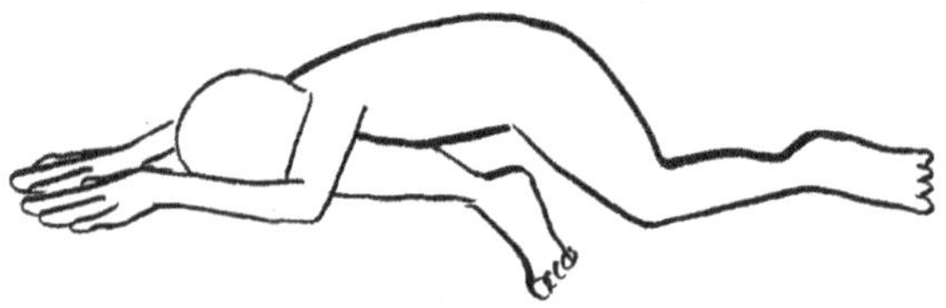

Gathering Breath

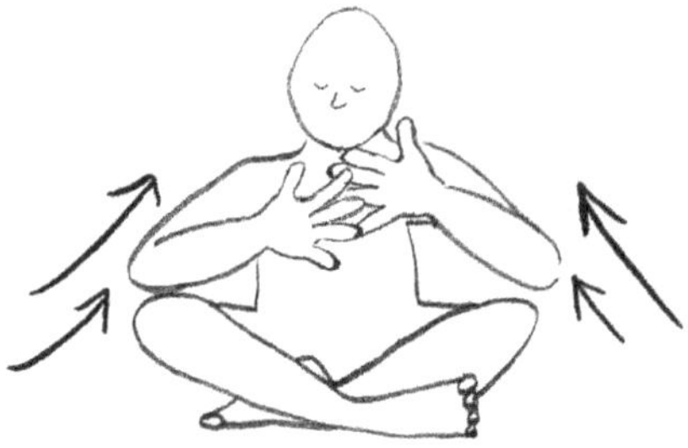

Child's Pose (cradling the face OR Inner Thigh Stretch)

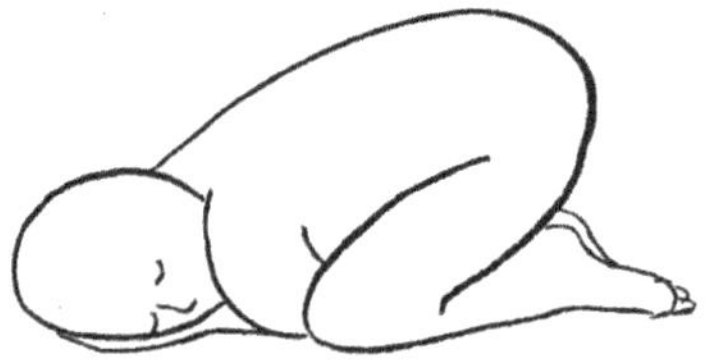

Wag the Dog's Tail

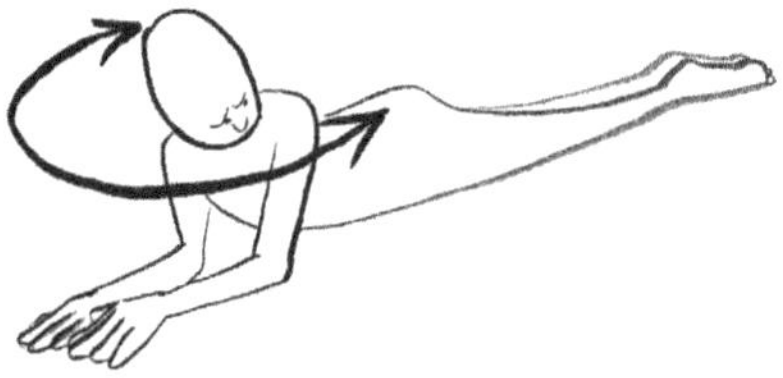

Diagonal Stretch

Cobra (3 of them)

Bend the Knees Circling

Turn the Head to One Side

Knees to Chest

Supine Hip Opener

Spinal Twist

Savasana

Testimonials

I just have to tell you that the training I took from you really transformed my practice and my teaching. What's really cool is seeing the transformation in my students who attend those classes. They love it! ~ Cindy F.

Your e-workbook is amazing. So well organized and full of great poses that aren't gymnastics disguised as yoga! Thank you so much. ~ Grace K.

Because I have only had experience with Hatha Yoga (also power yoga), I found this restorative form of yoga very soothing and energizing at the same time. I found myself connecting with my inner self in such a way that calmness did take me over. I learned to pay more attention to the littlest detail in my daily activities and everything that surrounds me. This training provided me with great ways on how to slow down my sometimes fast-paced life. The poses and movements were great in the sense that not much effort was needed to practice them. Yet, they were stimulating and refreshing. I would like for this training to take place in an outdoor type of setting where nature can play a role in this experience as well as adding more ways to develop or cultivate more awareness about our bodies, minds and surroundings (family, nature, work, etc.) I truly enjoyed the event, and I hope it happens again soon. ~ Leti G., Reynosa, Mexico

I began teaching a Restorative Flow class every Sat morning back in February, actually the weekend after I came to your training. It has been such a powerful pleasure for those that come. One of the women, Billye, had brain surgery in February and is very weak and shaky, and just is enjoying moving slowly and safely. Another, Kelly, who was coming before she was diagnosed with breast cancer is now recovering, having just finished chemo. These sweet women have been pretty ravaged. Both tell me again and again how much better, stronger, and encouraged they feel. I love what Restorative Flow does for people. I love it. I could teach it all the time. I cannot thank you enough for this gift to me and others. ~ Kathy C., yoga instructor, Texas

I really enjoyed the workshop and everyone participating. What a rich experience! So much stuff I can put to immediate use and allot of stuff to take in slowly... Everything about it was thought provoking and inspiring. ~ Ramona F., yoga instructor, Austin, Texas

Yoga should be accessible to everyone, and this style of yoga really allows all ages and abilities to benefit. And, yes, it is luxurious! ~ Tara M., yoga instructor, Dallas, Texas

Restorative Flow is a wonderfully gentle way to get to know your body. ~ Twila D., Austin, Texas

Learning Restorative Flow can make yoga classes inviting for all — not just the fitness enthusiasts, but for the people that have any limitations with their body. ~ Sue S., R.N., yoga instructor, Wisconsin

During my Monday morning class, I used several of the postures you provided to us and several of the cues and ideas incorporating the rocking motion. The class loved it and I got some really wonderful feedback afterward. The students are always complimentary, but that morning they were especially so. I truly feel it had to come from the new postures and ideas I received from your workshop. Thanks! ~ Cindy F. , San Antonio, Texas

The restorative flow yoga classes offer one's mind, body and spirit a gentle and beautiful invitation inward. ~ Jennifer H., Springfield, Virginia

The gift of Restorative Flow training is that it will not only enhance your yoga teaching skills, but you as a person. ~ Colleen H., yoga instructor, California

This style of yoga is particularly appropriate for those with disabilities and for caregiverse whose lives are shadowed by the constant needs of others. ~ Pat J., Stephenville, Texas

I love (and think everyone else did as well) the fabulously done Restorative Flow Teacher Training Workbook. it is thorough, concise and I especially like the illustrations. What a piece of work! And the restorative class itself peeled back many layers of stress in my body, mind and spirit. I believe this workshop is a valuable learning opportunity and covers a new approach to restorative yoga in detail, with humor, love and warmth. ~ Debbie C., yoga instructor, Bastrop, Texas

Restorative Flow is a gentle and affirming style of yoga. It is ideal for students who are new to yoga. ~ Jill F., yoga instructor at Women's Shelter, Pennsylvania

I love being able to use Restorative Flow with traditional hatha yoga. It makes it twice as valuable. It also gives me more confidence when working with students who have limited mobility. ~ Pam C., yoga instructor, Houston, Texas

During class I felt like I was a baby being swaddled in a mother's arms. ~ Jeannette Topica, Tulsa, Oklahoma

The workbook is excellent! I know I can use the material in my regular classes, or as a complete class by itself. ~ Corine Baerwald, yoga studio owner, Kerrville, Texas

As yoga students we are usually very impatient, and we think that classes should be harder and faster. I personally enjoy taking a restorative class. My body really appreciates it! ~ Luz B., yoga instructor, San Miguel, Mexico

The training and workbook gave me the confidence to start a Restorative Flow class, but also lots of ideas of poses and ways to teach that can be integrated into any class. ~ Gwynn G., yoga instructor, Kerrville, Texas

The longer I practice yoga the more I appreciate restorative poses. In this crazy fast paced world, they are invaluable! ~ Melodie W., yoga instructor, Austin, Texas

I loved this class and Donna's presentation. She projects such a calm and accepting presence that I feel instantly at east. She included visualization imagery with some movements; I responded deeply to these and liked the poses she chose. I also liked not doing imagery all the time. Donna's voice and pacing was wonderfully soothing. She gave very few verbal cues which helped me keep from thinking too much. The workbook has wonderful illustrations and directions, and I find it entirely user-friendly. Donna included brief meditations and ample break time, which kept me feeling relaxed; I did not feel hurried or "pushed." By serving us lunch at her studio on Saturday, we did not have to break the "spell" by getting out in traffic or deciding what and where to eat. Her studio and home are an excellent lo9cation for this type of training because it felt as if we were on a retreat rather than going to a teacher training workshop. I received excellent training and I'm sure I will use the restorative flow myself and hope to teach a restorative class someday. ~ Patti G., Texas